HOPE AND HEALING FOR FIBROMYALGIA WARRIORS

JAYDEN STEVE

COPYRIGHT

© 2024 by Jayden Steve

All rights reserved.

No part of this book may be reproduced, stored, or transmitted in any form or by any means, electronic, mechanical, photocopying, recording, scanning, or otherwise, without the prior written permission of the publisher, except for brief quotations in critical reviews or articles.

DEDICATION

To my fellow fibromyalgia warriors,

This book is dedicated to each one of you who bravely battles fibromyalgia every day. Your strength, resilience, and unwavering spirit inspire me and countless others on this journey. May this book serve as a beacon of hope, knowledge, and empowerment as we navigate the challenges of fibromyalgia together.

With love and solidarity,

Jayden Steve

TABLE OF CONTENT

COPYRIGHT 2

DEDICATION 3

CHAPTER ONE 9

INTRODUCTION TO FIBROMYALGIA 9

   UNDERSTANDING FIBROMYALGIA 11

   CAUSES AND TRIGGERS FOR FIBROMYALGIA 13

   THE COMMON MANIFESTATIONS OF FIBROMYALGIA 15

CHAPTER TWO 38

DIAGNOSIS OF 38

FIBROMYALGIA 38

   Differential Diagnosis 40

   Challenges in Diagnosis 44

CHAPTER THREE 48

CONVENTIONAL TREATMENTS FOR FIBROMYALGIA 48

Medications 48

- Analgesics and Nonsteroidal Anti-Inflammatory Drugs (NSAIDs) 49

- Antidepressants for Fibromyalgia 54

- Anticonvulsants for Fibromyalgia 58

- Muscle Relaxants for Fibromyalgia 61

- Utilizing Narcotics to Manage Pain 66

Doctors' Perspective on Prescription of Narcotics 69

Physical Therapy and Exercise 73

Guidelines for Optimal Stretching 90

- Cognitive-Behavioral Therapy (CBT) 96

- Mindfulness-Based Stress Reduction (MBSR) 107

- Relaxation Techniques 115

CHAPTER FOUR 123

ALTERNATIVE AND COMPLEMENTARY TREATMENTS 123

Acupuncture 123

Massage Therapy 133

Chiropractic Care 138

Dietary Supplements 143

Herbal remedies and flower essence 154

MIND-BODY PRACTICES 159

- YOGA FOR FIBROMYALGIA SUFFERERS 159

Tai Chi and Qigong 165

CHAPTER FIVE 179

LIFESTYLE MODIFICATIONS AND SELF-CARE 179

Diet and Nutrition 179

Sleep Hygiene 189

CHAPTER SIX 201

HELPFUL TIPS FOR FIBROMYALGIA PATIENTS 201

- Pain Prevention 201
- ☐ Managing Pain 203
- ☐ Getting the Sleep You Require 206
- ☐ Your Power Source 207
- ☐ Brain Fog 208

CHAPTER ONE

INTRODUCTION TO FIBROMYALGIA

In the quiet corners of my life, fibromyalgia became an uninvited companion, altering the landscape of my existence. Its arrival wasn't heralded with thunderous symptoms; instead, it crept in with persistent whispers of pain and fatigue. Each day felt like an intricate dance, navigating through a body that seemed to have its own rhythm, one filled with unpredictable highs and lows.

My journey with fibromyalgia has been a lesson in resilience and self-discovery. From the early days of confusion and misdiagnosis to the moments of clarity that came with understanding the condition, I learned to advocate for myself. It's a journey marked by small victories — the ability to find joy in simple pleasures, crafting a support system that understands the silent battles, and embracing a new normal.

Fibromyalgia has taught me the importance of pacing, the beauty of adapting, and the strength found in vulnerability. In the ebb and flow of symptoms, I've discovered an unwavering determination to savor life's moments, appreciating the strength that arises from adversity. My journey with fibromyalgia is not just a tale of pain; it's a narrative of resilience, courage, and the relentless pursuit of a life well-lived despite the challenges.

UNDERSTANDING FIBROMYALGIA

Fibromyalgia is a complex and often misunderstood chronic pain condition characterized by widespread musculoskeletal pain, tenderness, and fatigue. It is a disorder that affects the way the brain processes pain signals, leading to amplified pain sensations throughout the body. While the exact cause of fibromyalgia remains elusive, researchers believe it involves a combination of genetic, neurobiological, and environmental factors.

One of the defining features of fibromyalgia is the presence of tender points, which are specific areas on the body that are particularly sensitive to pressure. However, diagnosis is not solely based on tender points; it also involves a thorough assessment of symptoms and medical history. Common symptoms of fibromyalgia include chronic, widespread pain, fatigue, sleep disturbances, cognitive difficulties (often referred to as "fibro fog"), headaches, and mood disturbances such as anxiety and depression.

Fibromyalgia predominantly affects women, though it can occur in men and children as well. It can significantly impact an individual's quality of life, leading to physical limitations, emotional distress, and social isolation. Despite its prevalence and debilitating nature, fibromyalgia is often underdiagnosed or misdiagnosed due to the lack of specific diagnostic tests and the overlap of symptoms with other conditions.

CAUSES AND TRIGGERS FOR FIBROMYALGIA

The origins of fibromyalgia remain elusive, complicating the understanding of its causes. Genetic predispositions, however, play a role, as the condition tends to run in families. Environmental factors, such as infections or physical injuries, are considered potential triggers. Trauma, be it physical or emotional, is a noteworthy contributor; experiencing significant stress or undergoing surgeries may act as catalysts.

Neurochemical imbalances, particularly in neurotransmitters like serotonin and dopamine, are implicated in fibromyalgia. Abnormal pain perception, where the brain amplifies signals, contributes to the widespread discomfort characteristic of the condition. Hormonal imbalances, especially in relation to stress hormones, may also influence its onset and severity. Moreover, lifestyle factors, such as sedentary habits and poor sleep, can exacerbate symptoms. Weather changes, temperature extremes, and high humidity levels are reported as triggers by some individuals. Additionally, infections like the Epstein-Barr virus or Lyme disease have been associated with the development of fibromyalgia.

Understanding and managing fibromyalgia requires a holistic approach that acknowledges the interplay of genetic, environmental, and lifestyle factors. Identifying individual triggers is crucial for crafting personalized treatment plans and enhancing the overall well-being of those navigating the complex terrain of fibromyalgia.

THE COMMON MANIFESTATIONS OF FIBROMYALGIA

Here are some key symptoms individuals with fibromyalgia commonly experience:

- Chronic Pain

Chronic pain is the hallmark symptom of fibromyalgia. It typically manifests as widespread musculoskeletal pain, often described as a constant dull ache that affects multiple areas of the body. The pain may vary in intensity and can be exacerbated by physical activity, stress, weather changes, or lack of sleep. Common sites of pain include the neck, shoulders, back, hips, and extremities. Individuals with fibromyalgia may also experience heightened sensitivity to touch, known as allodynia, or increased pain perception to normal stimuli, referred to as hyperalgesia.

- Fatigue and Sleep Disturbances

Fatigue is another prevalent symptom of fibromyalgia, often described as overwhelming exhaustion that is not relieved by rest or sleep. Despite spending prolonged periods in bed, individuals with fibromyalgia may wake up feeling unrefreshed and continue to experience profound fatigue throughout the day. Sleep disturbances are common, including difficulty falling asleep, frequent awakenings, and non-restorative sleep patterns. Disrupted sleep can exacerbate fatigue and contribute to the overall burden of fibromyalgia symptoms.

- Cognitive Dysfunction (Fibro Fog)

Cognitive dysfunction, commonly referred to as "fibro fog," is a cognitive impairment that affects memory, concentration, and mental clarity in individuals with fibromyalgia. It is characterized by difficulty in processing information, short-term memory loss, word retrieval problems, and impaired focus and attention. Fibro fog can significantly impact daily functioning, leading to difficulties in performing tasks that require cognitive effort, such as work-related responsibilities, academic pursuits, or even engaging in conversations. The exact mechanisms underlying fibro fog are not fully understood but may involve disturbances in neurotransmitter levels and altered brain function.

• Other Associated Symptoms

In addition to the core symptoms mentioned above, individuals with fibromyalgia may experience a range of other associated symptoms, which can further contribute to the overall burden of the condition. These may include:
- Headaches:
 Chronic headaches, including tension-type headaches and migraines, are common among individuals with fibromyalgia and can significantly impact quality of life.
 - Irritable Bowel Syndrome (IBS):
Many individuals with fibromyalgia also experience gastrointestinal symptoms such as

abdominal pain, bloating, diarrhea, or constipation, which are characteristic of irritable bowel syndrome.

- Depression and Anxiety:

Fibromyalgia is often associated with mood disorders such as depression and anxiety, which may be both a consequence of living with chronic pain and a contributing factor to symptom exacerbation.

-Numbness and Tingling:

Some individuals with fibromyalgia may experience sensations of numbness, tingling, or burning in the extremities, known as paresthesia, which can occur spontaneously or in response to pressure or movement.

-Sensitivity to Environmental Stimuli:

Heightened sensitivity to light, sound, temperature, and odors is common in fibromyalgia and can exacerbate pain and discomfort.

Classifications of the different fibromyalgia symptoms:

GENERAL

1. The amount of activity dropped to less than 50% of what it was before sickness.
2. Cold digits (hands and feet)
3. Cough
4. A craving for starches(carbohydrates)
5. A delayed response to stressful situations or physical exertion
6. Dryness in the mouth or eyes
7. Swelling of hands and feet.
8. Relative(s) suffering from fibromyalgia
9. Fatigue exacerbated by physical activity or stress
10. Frequent chilly feelings
11. Frequent hot temperature
12. A lot of sighing
13. Palpitations in the heart
14. Rumbling in the throat

15. Hypoglycemia, or low blood sugar
16. Increased thirst
17. Low blood pressure (less than 110/70);
18. Inappropriately low body temperature (less than 97.6)
19. Fever of low grade
20. Sweats at night
21. Noisy joints, either painful or not
22. Inadequate blood flow to the hands and feet
23. Excessive perspiration 24. Recurrent feverish sickness
26. Severe nasal allergies (new or worsening allergies) 25. Shortness of breath with little to no exertion
27. Sore throat
28. Sensational edema in the extremities (feels bloated, although nothing is seen)
29. Perspiration
30. Symptoms made worse by flights

31. Stress-related worsening of symptoms

32. Temperature changes-related worsening of symptoms

33. Swollen or tender lymph nodes, particularly in the underarms and neck

34. Shuddering or quivering

35. Unexpected weight increase or decrease

36. Pain in the abdomen wall

37. Severe hip discomfort

38. Severe Neural Pain

39. Pain in the chest

40. Pain in the collarbone

41. Widespread edema

42. Pain in the elbow

43. Severe Plantar Arch or Heel Pain

44. "Growing" Pains that Persist After Growth

45. Tension or migraine Headache

46. Rigid Cartilage of the Ribs

47. Pain in the joints

48. Tender, lumpy breasts

49. Stiffness in the morning

51. Muscle spasms

50. Pain in the muscles

52. Spasticity of muscles

53. Weakness of muscles

54. Moderate to severe pain;

55. Pain that travels throughout the body;

56. Paralysis or extreme weakness in one or both arms or legs

57. Syndrome of Restless Legs

58. Pain in the ribs

59. Pain in the scalp (similar to hair pulling out)

60. Pain similar to sciatica

61. Points of tender or trigger

62. The ailment of TMJ

63. "Voodoo Doll" Prodding Feeling at Odd Locations

NEUROLOGICAL

64. Brain fog

65. Carpal tunnel syndrome

66 Blackouts

67. Experiential disorientation

68. Odor hallucinations

69. Difficulty to think clearly

70. Dizziness

71. Insensitivity to noise

72. Sensations of tingling or numbness

73. Light sensitivity, or photophobia

74. Convulsions

75. Incidents of seizures

76. Feeling as though you could pass out

Syncope (fainting): 77

78. Tinnitus, or ear ringing in either one or both

79. Dizziness or vertigo

EQUILIBRIUM/PERCEPTION

80. Running into objects
81. clumsy walking
82. Unable to Maintain Balance
83. Unable to judge distances (while driving, etc.)
84. Disorientation in direction
85. Dropping objects a lot
86. Experiencing spatial disorientation
87. Falling or tripping a lot
88. Not seeing what you're looking at
89. Having trouble with balance and coordination
90. An uneven gait

SLEEP

91. Energy and alertness peak late at night
92. Modified sleep/wake patterns
93. Frequent awakenings

94. Difficulty getting asleep

95. Difficulty staying asleep

96. Oversleeping

97. Abnormally high levels of alertness or energy at night

98. Dozing off at erratic and occasionally hazardous times

99. Weariness

100. Light or irregular sleep patterns

101. Nighttime twitches or spasms of the muscles

102. Narcolepsy

103. Disturbances in sleep

104. Feelings of falling or starting to sleep

105. Grinding of teeth

106. Turning over and tossing

107. Sleep that is neither restorative or rejuvenating

108. Detailed or upsetting dreams or nightmares

VISION/EYES

109. Visual blind spots;

110. Eye pain;

111. Trouble focusing on one item at a time;

112. Frequently fluctuating vision;

113. Difficulty driving at night

114. Occasionally blurry vision

115. Poor visibility at night

116. Vision that is rapidly deteriorating

117. Variations in vision

COGNITIVE

118. Getting lost while driving in familiar places

119. Being confused

120. Having trouble putting ideas into words

121. Finding it difficult to follow conversations, particularly when there is background noise

122. Inability to follow instructions when driving

123. Inability to follow spoken instructions

124. Having trouble adhering to written instructions
125. Difficulty making choices
126. Difficulty speaking
127. Difficulty focusing
128. Difficulty assembling thoughts into a coherent whole
129. Difficulty organizing tasks or objects in the right order
130 challenges such as facial recognition,
131 speaking unfamiliar words,
132 recalling object names,
133 recalling person names,
134 comprehension of what is read,
135 long-term memory problems.
136. Difficulty performing basic math
137. Short-term memory problems
138. Easily sidetracked when working on a task
139. Occasionally experiencing symptoms similar to dyslexia

140. Feeling too lost to drive

141. Forgetting how to execute simple tasks

142. Difficulty focusing;

143. Unable to identify familiar surroundings;

144. Losing focus mid-task (not remembering what to do next);

145. Divorcing your thoughts in the middle of a phrase; 146. Loss of color discrimination

147. Bad decision-making

148. Impaired short-term memory

149. Speaking more slowly

150. Staring off into space while attempting to think

151. Stuttering or stammering

152. Swapping back and forth

153. Reversing words, numbers, or letters while speaking

154. Reversing words, numbers, or letters when writing 155. Having trouble focusing

156. Using the incorrect term

157. Having trouble finding words Emotionally

158. Sudden and/or erratic mood changes 159. Outbursts of rage

160. Fear or anxiety when there is no apparent reason

161. Uncontrollably angry outbursts Reduced hunger

162, depressed mood

163, helplessness and/or hopelessness

164, fear of someone knocking on the door

165, fear of the phone ringing

166, feeling worthless

168, frequent crying

169, increased symptom awareness

170, incapacity to engage in previously enjoyed activities

171, irrational fears

172. Anger management

173. Exaggeration

174. Panic episodes

175. A change in personality is typically a worsening of a preexisting condition

176. Anxiety

177. Attempts at suicide

178. Suicidal ideation

179. Propensity to cry readily

GASTROINTESTINAL TRACT

180. Dizziness

181. Swelling

182. Diminished hunger

183. Cravings for food

184. Prolonged constipation

185. Consistent diarrhea

186. Symptoms similar to Gerd

187. Heartburn

(188). heightened hunger

189. Gas in the stomach

190. Irritable bowel syndrome

191. Nausea

192. Irritable bladder

193. Regurgitation

194. Stomach ache

195. throwing up

196. Gain in weight

197. Loss of weight

UROGENTAL

198. Reduced desire for sexual activity (libido)

199. Endometriosis

200. Prolonged urination

201. Impotence

202. Menstrual issues

203. Intractable bladder discomfort or painful urination
204. Pelvic pain
205. Prostate pain
206. Severe or worsening premenstrual syndrome (PMS)

SENSITIVITIES

207. Intolerance to alcohol
208. Hypersensitivity to touch (allodynia);
209. Modification of taste, smell, and/or hearing;
210. Sensitivity to chemicals found in fragrances, cleaning goods, and other items.
211. Food sensitivities
212. Light sensitivity;
213. Mold sensitivity;
214. Noise sensitivity;
215. Odor sensitivity; and

216. Yeast sensitivity (repeatedly developing yeast infections on skin, etc.)
217. Overloading the senses
218. Sensitivity to variations in humidity and pressure
219. Sensitivity to abrupt variations in temperature
220. Vulvodynia

SKIN

221. Capable of using finger to "write" on skin
222. Easily bruised
223. Bumpy and swollen
224. Psoriasis or eczema
225. Warm and dry skin
226. Hairs that grow back
227. Sensitivity to itching
228. Skin that is uneven
229. Skin irritations or sores
230. Easily scarring
231. Sun sensitivity

232. Reddening of the skin occurs abruptly

HEART-RELATED (CARDIOVASCULAR)

233. "click-murmur" sounds heard on stethoscope
234. An irregular pulse
235. Heart palpitations
236. An irregular pulse
237. An audible pulse in the ear
238. Differing pain from a heart attack
239. Fast heartbeat

NAILS AND HAIR

240. Lifeless, drab hair
241. Dense, split cuticles
242. irritated nail beds
243. Curving nails under
244. pronounced ridges on nails

245. momentary hair loss

OTHER

246. Canker sores 246; Dental issues 247; Disk Degeneration 248; Hemorrhoids 249; Nose bleedings 250

251. Gum disease, or periodontal disease

It is important to note that fibromyalgia is a heterogeneous condition, and not all individuals will experience the same combination or severity of symptoms. Furthermore, symptoms may overlap with those of other medical conditions, making accurate diagnosis and management essential. A multidisciplinary approach that addresses both physical and psychological aspects of fibromyalgia, including pharmacological interventions, lifestyle modifications, and complementary therapies, is often necessary to effectively manage symptoms and improve overall quality of life for individuals living with this challenging condition.

CHAPTER TWO
DIAGNOSIS OF FIBROMYALGIA

The diagnosis of fibromyalgia can be challenging due to the diverse range of symptoms and the absence of specific diagnostic tests. However, several criteria have been established to aid in the diagnosis of fibromyalgia. The most widely used criteria are those established by the American College of

Rheumatology (ACR) in 1990 and later revised in 2010.

According to the 2010 ACR criteria, a diagnosis of fibromyalgia can be made if the following conditions are met:

1. Widespread Pain: Pain must be present in all four quadrants of the body (i.e., both sides of the body and above and below the waist) for at least three months.

2. Tender Points: Presence of tenderness in at least 11 of 18 specified tender points when pressure is applied.

In addition to the ACR criteria, healthcare providers may also consider other factors such as the duration and severity of symptoms, the presence of other associated conditions, and the exclusion of alternative diagnoses.

It's important to note that while these criteria provide a framework for diagnosis, fibromyalgia remains a clinical diagnosis, and healthcare providers may use their discretion in interpreting and applying these criteria based on individual patient presentations.

Differential Diagnosis

Diagnosing fibromyalgia requires careful consideration of various factors due to its overlapping symptoms with many other medical conditions. Here are some of the key differential diagnoses healthcare providers consider when evaluating a patient with symptoms suggestive of fibromyalgia:

1. Rheumatoid Arthritis (RA) and Other Inflammatory Arthropathies:

Conditions such as rheumatoid arthritis, systemic lupus erythematosus (SLE), and other autoimmune diseases can cause widespread joint pain, fatigue, and stiffness, similar to fibromyalgia. However, these conditions often present with additional symptoms such as joint swelling, inflammation, and elevated inflammatory markers in blood tests.

2. Chronic Fatigue Syndrome (CFS):

Chronic fatigue syndrome shares many symptoms with fibromyalgia, including profound fatigue, sleep disturbances, and cognitive difficulties. However, while pain is a primary feature of fibromyalgia, it is not a defining criterion for CFS. Additionally, individuals with CFS may experience more pronounced post-exertional malaise and flu-like symptoms.

3. Hypothyroidism:

Thyroid disorders, particularly hypothyroidism, can cause symptoms such as fatigue, muscle pain, and cognitive impairment that overlap with fibromyalgia. Blood tests measuring thyroid hormone levels can help differentiate between these conditions.

4. Myofascial Pain Syndrome (MPS):

Myofascial pain syndrome is characterized by localized areas of muscle pain and tenderness, known as trigger points, which can mimic the tender points seen in fibromyalgia. However, MPS typically involves specific muscle groups rather than the widespread pain distribution seen in fibromyalgia.

5. Depression and Anxiety Disorders:

Mood disorders such as depression and anxiety commonly coexist with fibromyalgia and can exacerbate its symptoms. While these conditions may share symptoms such as fatigue and sleep disturbances, they are distinct diagnoses that require separate evaluation and management.

6. Multiple Sclerosis (MS):

Multiple sclerosis is a neurological disorder that can cause widespread pain, fatigue, and cognitive dysfunction similar to fibromyalgia. However, MS is characterized by additional neurological symptoms such as weakness, sensory disturbances, and visual changes, which are not typically seen in fibromyalgia.

Distinguishing fibromyalgia from these and other potential differential diagnoses requires a thorough medical history, physical examination, and, in some cases, laboratory tests and imaging studies. Collaboration between healthcare providers from various specialties may be necessary to accurately diagnose and manage patients with suspected fibromyalgia.

Challenges in Diagnosis

Diagnosing fibromyalgia poses several challenges for both patients and healthcare providers due to the complexity of its symptoms and the lack of specific diagnostic tests. Some of the primary challenges in diagnosing fibromyalgia include:

1. Subjectivity of Symptoms:

Fibromyalgia symptoms such as pain, fatigue, and cognitive dysfunction are subjective and can vary widely among individuals. This variability makes it challenging to establish a standardized diagnostic framework and can lead to inconsistencies in diagnosis between healthcare providers.

2. Overlap with Other Conditions:

Fibromyalgia shares symptoms with many other medical conditions, including rheumatoid arthritis, lupus, chronic fatigue syndrome, and mood disorders such as depression and anxiety. The overlap in symptoms can make it difficult to differentiate fibromyalgia from other conditions, leading to misdiagnosis or delayed diagnosis.

3. Absence of Specific Biomarkers:

Unlike many other chronic conditions, fibromyalgia lacks specific biomarkers or laboratory tests for definitive diagnosis. While imaging studies and blood tests may be used to rule out other conditions, there are no tests that can confirm the presence of fibromyalgia itself. This absence of objective markers can contribute to diagnostic uncertainty and skepticism among some healthcare providers.

4. Diagnostic Criteria Limitations:

Although diagnostic criteria such as the American College of Rheumatology (ACR) criteria provide guidelines for diagnosing fibromyalgia, they have limitations. For example, the tender point criterion in the previous ACR criteria has been criticized for its subjectivity and lack of sensitivity. The revised 2010 ACR criteria, which focus more on widespread pain and symptom severity, have improved diagnostic accuracy but may still miss cases of fibromyalgia with atypical presentations.

5. Patient Advocacy and Stigma:

Many individuals with fibromyalgia face challenges in having their symptoms taken seriously by healthcare providers. Due to the lack of objective diagnostic markers and the subjective nature of symptoms, some patients may encounter skepticism, dismissiveness, or even accusations of malingering. This lack of validation can exacerbate the psychological distress associated with fibromyalgia and delay diagnosis and treatment.

In summary, the challenges in diagnosing fibromyalgia underscore the need for increased awareness, improved diagnostic criteria, and a patient-centered approach that acknowledges the complex interplay of physical, psychological, and social factors in this condition. By addressing these challenges, healthcare providers can enhance early detection and facilitate timely intervention for individuals living with fibromyalgia.

CHAPTER THREE

CONVENTIONAL TREATMENTS FOR FIBROMYALGIA

Medications

To help you manage the aching, stiffness, and general pain of fibromyalgia, your doctor may prescribe painkillers or other kinds of treatments.

If your symptoms have partly subsided but you still feel like you could use some pain relief, an over-the-counter pain reliever could be the best option for you. I go over some of the alternatives in the sections that follow.

- **Analgesics and Nonsteroidal Anti-Inflammatory Drugs (NSAIDs)**

Analgesics and Nonsteroidal Anti-Inflammatory Drugs (NSAIDs) are commonly used medications in managing fibromyalgia symptoms, particularly pain and inflammation. Here's an overview of how they work, their pros and cons, and cautions for their use, along with some examples of each:

How They Work:

Analgesics:

Analgesics are medications primarily designed to relieve pain. They work by inhibiting pain signals sent to the brain or by reducing the brain's perception of pain. Common analgesics used in fibromyalgia management include acetaminophen (Tylenol) and opioid medications such as tramadol (Ultram). Acetaminophen works centrally in the brain to reduce pain perception, while opioids act on opioid receptors in the brain and spinal cord to block pain signals.

Nonsteroidal Anti-Inflammatory Drugs (NSAIDs):

NSAIDs work by inhibiting the activity of cyclooxygenase (COX) enzymes, which are involved in the production of prostaglandins—chemicals that promote inflammation, pain, and fever. By reducing prostaglandin levels, NSAIDs help alleviate pain and inflammation associated with conditions like fibromyalgia. Common NSAIDs include ibuprofen (Advil, Motrin), naproxen (Aleve), and aspirin.

Pros:

Pain Relief:

Both analgesics and NSAIDs can provide effective pain relief for individuals with fibromyalgia, helping to improve overall quality of life.

Readily Available:

Many analgesics and NSAIDs are available over the counter, making them easily accessible for symptom management.

Variety of Options: There are various types of analgesics and NSAIDs available, allowing for flexibility in finding the most effective medication for each individual.

Cons and Cautions:

Side Effects:

Analgesics and NSAIDs can cause side effects such as gastrointestinal irritation, ulcers, kidney problems, and liver damage, particularly with long-term use or high doses.

Risk of Dependence:

Opioid analgesics, in particular, carry a risk of dependence and addiction, making them unsuitable for long-term use in most cases.

Interaction with Other Medications:

NSAIDs can interact with other medications, including blood thinners and certain antidepressants, increasing the risk of side effects or reducing effectiveness.

Examples:

Analgesics:

Acetaminophen (Tylenol), tramadol (Ultram)

NSAIDs:

Ibuprofen (Advil, Motrin), naproxen (Aleve), aspirin.

When given topically to the muscle, nonsteroidal anti-inflammatory drugs (NSAIDs) can be quite efficient at relieving fibromyalgia pain because they penetrate the muscle tissue (Yunus 1989). When applied topically as opposed to orally, NSAIDs are found in muscle tissue at a concentration four to seven times higher (Tegeder 1999; Dominkus 1996). Furthermore, topical NSAIDs have fewer dangers than oral ones since relatively little of them enter the bloodstream, despite the fact that oral NSAIDs can irritate the stomach lining and cause additional side effects (Heyneman 2000). In Europe, topical NSAIDs are frequently sold over-the-counter and have been used for a long time. In the US, there are three prescription formulations available. Even though the FDA only permits their usage for knee and hand pain associated with osteoarthritis, they might be beneficial on any localized area of muscle or fascial

• Antidepressants for Fibromyalgia

Antidepressants are commonly used in the management of fibromyalgia due to their ability to alleviate pain, improve sleep quality, and address mood disturbances associated with the condition. While fibromyalgia is not primarily a mental health disorder, antidepressants have demonstrated efficacy in treating its symptoms, suggesting a complex interplay between pain perception, mood regulation, and neurotransmitter function.

Antidepressants used for fibromyalgia include selective serotonin reuptake inhibitors (SSRIs), serotonin-norepinephrine reuptake inhibitors (SNRIs), and tricyclic antidepressants (TCAs). Duloxetine (Cymbalta) and milnacipran (Savella) are FDA-approved SNRIs for fibromyalgia, while TCAs like amitriptyline and nortriptyline are also commonly prescribed off-label.

These antidepressants work by modulating the levels of neurotransmitters in the brain, particularly serotonin and norepinephrine, which are involved in regulating pain perception, mood, and sleep. By increasing the availability of these neurotransmitters in the brain, antidepressants may help reduce pain sensitivity, improve mood, and promote better sleep quality in individuals with fibromyalgia.

Pros of using antidepressants for fibromyalgia include:

1. Pain Relief: Antidepressants can help alleviate both musculoskeletal and neuropathic pain associated with fibromyalgia.

2. Improved Sleep: By enhancing serotonin and norepinephrine activity, antidepressants may aid in improving sleep quality and reducing sleep disturbances.

3. Mood Stabilization: Antidepressants can address mood symptoms such as depression and anxiety, which commonly coexist with fibromyalgia.

4. Non-habit forming: Unlike opioid medications, antidepressants are not habit-forming and carry a lower risk of dependence.

However, there are some cons and cautions to consider when using antidepressants for fibromyalgia:

1. Side Effects: Common side effects of antidepressants include nausea, dizziness, dry mouth, constipation, and weight changes.

2. Adjustment Period: It may take several weeks for the full therapeutic effects of antidepressants to be felt, and dosage adjustments may be necessary to achieve optimal symptom relief.

3. Drug Interactions: Antidepressants can interact with other medications, so it's important to inform your healthcare provider about all medications you're taking.

4. Withdrawal Symptoms: Abruptly discontinuing antidepressants can lead to withdrawal symptoms, so it's essential to taper off them under medical supervision.

Most rheumatologists occasionally give their fibromyalgia patients two antidepressants at the same time in the hopes that they may experience more alleviation. For instance, fibromyalgia patients in one research trial received both Elavil (25 mg) and 20 milligrams of Prozac. As a result, a sizable amount of patients experienced twice as much pain relief from this combination than with either medication alone. Despite your innate belief that taking two medications would logically provide you with roughly twice the alleviation that you would from taking one, this result is uncommon.

- **Anticonvulsants for Fibromyalgia**

Anticonvulsants, originally developed to treat epilepsy, have gained popularity in managing fibromyalgia symptoms due to their ability to modulate pain signals in the central nervous system. While not fully understood, their effectiveness in fibromyalgia is believed to be linked to their ability to stabilize abnormal electrical activity in the brain, reducing the sensitivity of pain-processing neurons and improving pain thresholds.

Anticonvulsive medications are used by certain doctors to treat FMS patients for pain and tenderness, even if the patients have never experienced a seizure. Anticonvulsives are an excellent means of reducing anxiety and calming hyperactive pain fibers. To be certain if a medication is effective, you have to take it and observe how it affects you.

Anticonvulsants such as pregabalin (Lyrica) and gabapentin (Neurontin) are commonly prescribed for fibromyalgia. These medications work by binding to calcium channels in the central nervous system, reducing the release of neurotransmitters involved in pain transmission. By dampening nerve excitability, they can alleviate neuropathic pain, muscle spasms, and sleep disturbances associated with fibromyalgia.

One of the main advantages of anticonvulsants in fibromyalgia management is their ability to address multiple symptoms simultaneously. In addition to pain relief, they can improve sleep quality, reduce fatigue, and enhance overall functioning. Unlike opioids, they are not associated with the risk of addiction or tolerance development, making them safer for long-term use.

However, anticonvulsants may also have some drawbacks. Common side effects include dizziness, drowsiness, weight gain, and cognitive impairment, which can limit their tolerability and adherence. Additionally, discontinuation of these medications may lead to withdrawal symptoms in some individuals. There is also a potential for drug interactions with other medications, necessitating careful monitoring when used in combination therapy.

When managing fibromyalgia with anticonvulsants, healthcare providers should exercise caution, especially in vulnerable populations such as older adults and those with preexisting medical conditions. Starting with low doses and gradually titrating upward can help minimize side effects and improve tolerability. Regular monitoring for adverse effects and therapeutic efficacy is essential to optimize treatment outcomes.

- **Muscle Relaxants for Fibromyalgia**

Muscle relaxants are a class of medications commonly used in the management of fibromyalgia to alleviate muscle pain, stiffness, and spasms. While not specifically approved by the FDA for fibromyalgia treatment, muscle relaxants are often prescribed off-label to address the musculoskeletal symptoms associated with the condition.

Why Muscle Relaxants are Used in Fibromyalgia: Muscle relaxants are utilized in fibromyalgia treatment to target the muscular component of the condition. Fibromyalgia is characterized by widespread musculoskeletal pain and tenderness, often accompanied by muscle stiffness and spasms. Muscle relaxants work by dampening excessive muscle activity, reducing tension, and promoting relaxation, which can help alleviate pain and improve overall function.

How Muscle Relaxants Work:

Muscle relaxants exert their effects by acting on the central nervous system, primarily targeting the brain and spinal cord. They typically work by enhancing the inhibitory neurotransmitter gamma-aminobutyric acid (GABA) or blocking excitatory signals within the nervous system. By modulating neural activity, muscle relaxants help reduce muscle tone and promote muscle relaxation, thereby alleviating pain and stiffness associated with fibromyalgia.

Pros and Cons of Muscle Relaxants:

Pros:

- Effective in reducing muscle pain, stiffness, and spasms.

- Can improve sleep quality by promoting muscle relaxation.

- May complement other fibromyalgia treatments, such as exercise and physical therapy.
- Generally well-tolerated when used as directed.

Cons:
- Potential side effects, including drowsiness, dizziness, and fatigue, which may impair daily functioning.
- Risk of dependence or tolerance with long-term use.
- Not suitable for everyone, particularly individuals with certain medical conditions or those taking other medications.
- Limited evidence supporting their efficacy specifically for fibromyalgia.

Cautions for Managing Fibromyalgia with Muscle Relaxants (with Drug Examples):

When using muscle relaxants for fibromyalgia management, it's essential to exercise caution and follow healthcare provider recommendations. Some key considerations include:

- Starting with a low dose and gradually titrating upward to minimize side effects.
- Avoiding concurrent use of alcohol or other central nervous system depressants, which can potentiate sedative effects.
- Monitoring for potential adverse reactions and adjusting treatment as needed.
- Discussing potential drug interactions with healthcare providers, especially if taking other medications concurrently.

Common muscle relaxants used in fibromyalgia management include cyclobenzaprine (Flexeril), tizanidine (Zanaflex), and baclofen (Lioresal). These medications may be prescribed alone or in combination with other therapies as part of a comprehensive treatment approach for fibromyalgia.

• Utilizing Narcotics to Manage Pain

It is up to you and your doctor to decide whether or not to use opioids in your pain management regimen. Narcotics can reduce moderate to severe pain when recommended for those with chronic pain, improving the patient's quality of life. Being in constant discomfort as a sufferer, you ought to be given the option of using this or not.

Before thinking about using drugs, patients with FM should be aware of the following three facts:

1. Narcotics are strong, perhaps addictive substances.

2. The majority of individuals with chronic pain do not develop a narcotics addiction, as addiction is mostly governed by biological factors.

3. If you have persistent pain, narcotics can be your only option for relief.

Physicians must abide by FDA restrictions when writing prescriptions for opioids. You should understand the difference between narcotics used as recreational drugs and narcotics used as chronic pain treatment before making your own decisions regarding them. Because narcotics can make some people feel euphoric, they are abused as recreational substances. For instance, oxycontin has gained widespread recognition as a street drug. Drug addicts can easily obtain it, and it produces a potent, long-lasting euphoric impact.

Narcotics are not taken by drug abusers as directed. The specific medication's dosage instructions, which can be given orally, as an intravenous, liquid, or through a skin patch, will be specified in a prescription. Narcotics are broken up and snorted into the nose when taken as street drugs, which gives consumers a stronger, more intense concentration and a quicker effect.

The euphoric benefits of opioids are rare for individuals with chronic pain, and only a small proportion of these patients ever develop an addiction. Dr. James J. Holman agrees, saying that it's interesting that the majority of patients with FM encounter numerous adverse drug reactions. Describe a group that refuses to take any medication. Hence, the queries about addiction are a little absurd. Sandra W. of Seattle was inundated with worried relatives and friends who questioned her use of the opioid methadone after she was prescribed it. However, Sandra saw methadone as a step toward a life free from FM discomfort: "It was pretty amazing not to have to deal with pain every day when I woke up in the morning."

I felt so strongly about it. Before, even though my ex-husband doesn't even take aspirin, I detested having to take medicine and the idea that he would label me a drug addict. As a result, I also had to cope with stigma—people judging my actions and my body's worth. Methadone has made it possible for me to function. Sandra wishes to make it clear to those who would label her a drug addict: "I get hope on methadone; I don't get high."

Doctors' Perspective on Prescription of Narcotics

For a number of reasons, including lack of experience treating chronic pain and concern of creating addiction, doctors are hesitant to prescribe opiates for long-term pain, including constipation, lethargy, and respiratory issues. Of course, losing one's license is a more urgent concern. The views of medical disciplinary bodies are ones of fear.

Physicians who continue to prescribe drugs for the treatment of chronic nonmalignant pain run the danger of facing sanctions and restrictions from their medical board. This is a belief shared by many doctors. Losing the capacity to practice is the practical result of any limitation, which is the board's minimal action.

For the sake of relieving pain, the majority of doctors are unwilling to take the chance of losing their license.

America was unprepared for the Oxycontin crisis, which resulted in stricter guidelines for the prescription of Schedule II drugs. Similarly, the problem of managing pain has been made worse by the fall in the widespread usage of COX inhibitors like Bextra and Vioxx due to concerns that these drugs raise the risk of cardiovascular disease. The lesson from Vioxx appears to be that, even in cases when a medication proves to be beneficial, access to it may be swiftly restricted because to concerns about product liability and litigation.

Even though there is very little chance of addiction in patients with chronic pain, many doctors are still reluctant to take the chance.

Although the exact percentage of the general population at risk for opiate addiction is unknown, it is undoubtedly less than 10%. Asking the following question can help to illustrate the treatment dilemma: For every ten patients who present with chronic, intractable pain that does not improve with non-opioid treatment, there is a 10% chance that they may become addicted to opiates. Is it moral to deny treatment to the other nine individuals in case one of them develops an addiction to the medication in order to prevent the one from becoming addicted? When you take into account that the actual risk is far less than 10 percent, I think the answer to that question is "No," and an even stronger "NO!" For chronic, nonmalignant pain, narcotic analgesics—like oxycodone—have been shown to be a reliable and efficient treatment. I've provided care for individuals whose chronic pain has rendered them unable of carrying out daily tasks, much less working. By taking prescribed amounts of opioids responsibly, these same people have successfully resumed their jobs and found happiness in their lives again without experiencing any negative side effects. They are not addicted or have tolerance, thus they can continue taking prescribed dosages. Research has shown that there is little chance of addiction while treating chronic pain. In a collaborative pharmacological research conducted in Boston, out of 11,882 individuals treated with opiates, only 4 developed an addiction. Not one of the 10,000 patients treated at national burn clinics developed an addiction. Just three of the 2,369 individuals who received treatment for migraines developed an addiction.

For chronic, nonmalignant pain, narcotic analgesics—like oxycodone—have been shown to be a reliable and efficient treatment. I've provided care for those who've

Physical Therapy and Exercise

Many individuals have the misconception that exercising makes fibromyalgia sufferers worse off and is not recommended for them.

Exercise itself isn't the issue, though. It's the kind of exercise that individuals are engaging in.

According to Mously LeBlanc, MD, "exercise-related pain is very common with fibromyalgia." "Exercising appropriately can help improve symptoms; it's not about exercising hard, which causes significant pain", its about exercising appropriately to help improve symptoms.

She also tells Healthline that maintaining a regular physical exercise schedule is essential for fibromyalgia sufferers to get the best possible pain relief.

Expert on fibromyalgia Dr. Jacob Teitelbaum claims that overexertion during exercise is the cause of the "post-exertional malaise" difficulties that many encounter after working out.

He claims that this happens because fibromyalgia sufferers lack the energy to condition in comparison to those who can manage the increase in exercise and conditioning.

- Aerobic Exercises

Numerous studies have demonstrated that fibromyalgia sufferers who engage in regular aerobic exercise experience improvements in pain, function, and general quality of life.

Gentle aerobic exercise is often advised as the initial course of treatment for fibromyalgia by medical professionals. This is prior to the consideration of any kind of medication. It's crucial to stay active even if your doctor prescribes medicine for your illness.

Less time spent sitting and more modest physical activity was linked to decreased discomfort, exhaustion, and the overall burden of the condition in one study involving over 400 women (Trusted Source).

If you're too exhausted or it hurts too much to work out, you might start with mild exercises like walking or swimming. You can gradually increase your strength and endurance if you do this on a regular basis.

Gradually increasing aerobic exercise under prescription is a successful treatment for fibromyalgia patients that improves their self-reported health. Engaging in an activity that elevates your heart rate and keeps it elevated for a prolonged amount of time is called aerobic exercise. The health guidelines recommend aerobic exercise at least three times a week, with an intensity of between 60% and 70% of your age-predicted maximal heart rate (anything above this may be overdoing it). The heart rate at which you should be exercising is 60% to 70% of your age-predicted heart rate, which is calculated by deducting your age from 220. A woman in her 40s, for instance, might figure out the following:

Calculating Your Heart Rate Based on Your Age
Her maximal heart rate was 220 - 40 = 180.
60% x 180 = 108 beats per minute is the calculation.
70% x 180 = 126 beats per minute is the calculation.
She should aim for a heart rate in the range of 108 to 126 beats per minute.

It may be necessary for people with FM to start at the lower end of this heart rate range, if not much lower.

Because aerobic exercise releases endogenous endorphins, which are compounds that resemble hormones, it can also improve psychological well-being, self-efficacy, and pain alleviation. These compounds function as analgesics because they bind to particular opiate receptors in the brain to either block or regulate pain originating from the musculoskeletal system. This is known by some experts as the "runner's high."

Begin with a low-impact exercise like swimming, walking, cycling, or using a treadmill. One to three days following exercise, pain may manifest. This is why you should only intensify your routine once a week so that you may continue to pay attention to your body and its responses. When you begin a new program, it is typical to experience some discomfort, or tightness in your muscles. However, intense pain is a sign that you have most likely overexercised your muscles. Recognize your body's needs and refrain from pushing yourself to achieve unattainable objectives. It will be up to you to decide when enough is enough. Pay attention to your gut. Nobody is better than u at differentiating your agony.

Before beginning a jogging or other "high-impact" exercise program, if you were an athlete prior to the onset of FM, you should consult your doctor to assess the benefits and suitability of the activity. It has been observed that high-impact activity exacerbates FM symptoms.

It should get more and more comfortable as your tolerance for activity rises. It is crucial to keep in mind that frequent exercise is necessary for it to be beneficial. It is usually advised to engage in aerobic activity for 20 to 30 minutes. If you do not experience any worsening of your discomfort, try to progressively increase your weekly exercise time to 40 or even 60 minutes three times a week. You might need to start out exercising for as little as five to ten minutes at a time. You must calm down and give your immune system time to function, even if it may be difficult if you have always led a busy lifestyle. Once more, treat yourself to something for every bit of activity you manage. To ensure that you complete your program, look for support networks.

Your objective is to safely begin, continue, and/or enhance your exercise routine.

Walking:

You may need to start off very gently if you haven't included walking in your aerobics program for a time (generally, three to six months). On the first day, just walk for five minutes. Add one minute to this sum the next day. Until you are walking for thirty minutes, keep adding one or two minutes each day.

Certain medical professionals advise increasing the amount of exercise by no more than 10% every week. Put otherwise, if you can initially walk for only five minutes, then aim for only thirty seconds more during the second week. You'll need to ascertain what is appropriate for you and what your upper bound is.

Walk three or four times a week once you've reached the stage where you're doing it for at least thirty to one hour. If you are having trouble expanding the length of your walk from thirty minutes, stick to what is comfortable for you. For several days or for however long is necessary, remain at that amount of time. Until you accomplish your goal, keep adding minutes to the total. Walking will make you feel accomplished since you are managing your pain and fatigue and building muscle strength, even though it won't cure fibromyalgia.

No matter how long or how far you walk, give yourself credit for it.

Walking-to-jogging routines:

After you feel comfortable walking three or four times a week, you can alternate between walking and slow jogging for younger people who want a more intense workout than walking may offer. Go for a two-block stroll followed by a one-block jog; repeat this pattern for another two blocks. As long as it feels comfortable, continue doing this. As part of your warm-up and cool-down, start and finish your workout with just walking. Given that jogging is a high-impact workout, be sure that doing so won't make your symptoms worse.

Cycling:

One advantage of stationary bikes, often known as exercise bikes, is that you can work out indoors. Riding a bicycle outside provides fresh air, which might enhance one's sense of wellbeing, for those who can manage it. Track your distance or aim to ride your bike for 15 to 30 minutes each day. After stretching, begin pedaling for five minutes at a time and work your way up to roughly twenty. For those with FM, riding upright or in a recumbent position tends to be less stressful. It might not be as pleasant to ride a bicycle in the forward-bent position used by professional cyclists. Always remember to warm up and cool down before beginning any program.

Water aerobics:

Both people who can swim and those who can't benefit greatly from water/aquatic exercise. First off, the majority of the body floats in the water, which lessens the force of gravity on joints and muscles. The majority of pools are maintained at temperatures below 85°F; still, a temperature between 88° and 90°F will help to better relax muscles and facilitate easier stretching. Hot tubs or warm-water spas can be found in some fitness centers or rehabilitative clinics..

All of your major muscle groups must be used, whether you are swimming or other in-place water aquatic exercises. Always remember to warm up and cool down before beginning any program.

For non-swimmers:

At first, range of motion, flexibility, strengthening, and cardio workouts can be supervised by a qualified specialist. You can perform all of these in the water. You can follow your own program by yourself or with other people once you're comfortable doing so. With an Aquajogger or other flotation device that fastens over your chest, you can push against the water's resistance by standing in a swimming pool and walking or "running." Work out your lower extremities with a kickboard.

For swimmers:
Practice crawling or freestyle for five to ten minutes, followed by five minutes of backstroke. Your shoulder muscles will be stretched and relaxed as a result. Your chest muscles will be stretched by doing a breaststroke for five to ten minutes. Change up your practice by employing varied arm strokes and kicks based on what is bearable if your hips are hurting.

Taking a walk:
You can create a home workout regimen with the assistance of a physical therapist, but why not start with just walking? The best forms of activities are frequently the most basic.

All you need is a good pair of shoes, and you can perform it anyplace. Walk for shorter distances at a leisurely pace at first, then increase to longer walks. The Mayo Clinic suggests that working up to at least 30 minutes of aerobic activity three times a week is a desirable goal.

Pool workouts

A gentle workout combined with warm water can help reduce the pain associated with fibromyalgia. Activity in a pool was superior to aerobic activity in the gym or stretching and strengthening exercises performed at home for the relief of fibromyalgia symptoms, according to research on women between the ages of 18 and 50.

Stretching

Stretching can assist with reversing FM's overall lack of flexibility. Maintaining the length and strength of the soft tissue around a joint (such as the capsule and ligaments) and allowing the joint to move through its entire range of motion can help to preserve the nutrients that the synovial joints' cartilage receives. You run the risk of losing range of motion if you don't stretch frequently. For instance, the muscles that move the joint start to atrophy and the connective tissues around the joint start to alter practically quickly following hospitalization and/or surgery. The ensuing physiological repercussions cause these structures to shorten, which depletes the joint's nutrition and prolongs the joint's range of motion.

Although many sources recommend stretching before warm-up, it's actually safer to stretch after a brief period of both the warm-up and warm-down (cool-down) from the cardiovascular exercise. Stretching muscles and tendons is made easier by warming up. Stretching is said by many to help lower the risk of muscle injury; also, if you do not warm up before doing out, you may feel more pain, burning, and cramping. Some sources, however, assert that overstretching—unless it's for gymnastics, dance, or sprinting—may potentially increase the risk of injury. You will need to determine your course of action in consultation with your personal physician, physical therapist, or trainer.

You might not be able to hold a stretch for longer than a few seconds at first. Every accomplishment counts, and you'll make more progress more quickly if you're patient. Acknowledge from away that this is a gradual process, but that perseverance and commitment to work out will pay off handsomely, teaching you valuable things about how your body works and what kinds of activities it can perform.

You should be able to conduct some safe flexibility exercises if you are unable to choose an aerobic (cardiovascular) routine. Some of these need someone else to help you, and stretching frequently needs to be done after taking some medicine. Stretching for a few days should definitely be the first step in any workout regimen, even for those who are just starting out. This is how you start for two reasons:

Since most exercise programs include flexibility exercises as part of their warm-up and cool-down, it is imperative that you learn them. Additionally, a large portion of FM discomfort is related to the muscles and tendons, which connect the muscle to the bone. These structures typically become shorter as people age and can cause pain or discomfort when they are stretched or constricted, which is what most workout regimens do.

Self-stretch and assisted stretch are the two forms of stretching. There are a variety of self-stretch regimens available; it is advisable to consult a qualified healthcare professional to determine the most suitable one. Almost all self-stretch exercises require the practice of mental relaxation and breathing control to ensure that the breath is released evenly and slowly. Stretching that is assisted is done in a group setting, either at home or in a professional's office.

Guidelines for Optimal Stretching

1. It is normally best to stretch after both the warm-up and the warm-down (cool-down). Avoid stretching yourself cold!

2. Stretching that is static or prolonged ought to be limited to what is comfortable. Stretch in a single direction gently and steadily. For at least five to six seconds, hold the stretch.

3. Don't forget to breathe consistently. Regularly and deeply inhale. Inhale through your nose, then exhale through tightly closed lips.

4. Work your way up to 5 to 10 repetitions (or "reps") of each exercise starting with 1 to 3.

5. Use softer movements and fewer repetitions if a particular muscle or joint is particularly sore on a given day.

6. Stretch the main muscle groups gently for a duration of 5 to 10 seconds. Taking it slowly could help you avoid cramping.

7. Muscle stretches easier when done in warm water, like in a shower or whirlpool.

It's important to always stretch slowly. Dynamic, rhythmic bouncing exercises at the limit of a muscle's range of motion are called ballistic stretching. It is not advisable to do ballistic stretching since this rapid, high-impact motion could injure your muscles.

Preventing muscle tightness and stiffness during the day can be achieved by performing stretching exercises. Include exercise in everyday tasks like making the bed or cleaning the dishes, as well as in between periods of immobile work like typing or reading.

Don't miss your warm-up if you just have a short window of time for aerobic activity on some days.

On those days, if necessary, cut the aerobic portion of the workout short.

Strength exercises

Acute and chronic fatigue sufferers should be encouraged to understand that they can progressively increase their exercise if they are patient, even if they are unable to conduct strength (resistance) training at certain points in their programs.

Physical therapists use wide, different-colored elastic bands to gradually strengthen muscles. Sports retailers sell these for a reasonable price as well. To avoid hurting joints, it's crucial to work with these in gentle, steady motions.

Weight training and other resistance exercise offer several advantages to anyone who can extend their program duration and stamina to incorporate this kind of physical activity. Resistance training has a number of general health benefits, including protecting the lower back and weak joints and slowing the osteoporosis-related bone loss. It also increases muscle strength.

Lifting or pushing a weight against gravity and repeating the motion several times (also known as repetitions or "reps") is the norm for strength training. The degree of effort required for the exercise is determined by the weight and repetition count. When doing the lift (or push), exhale during the major effort and inhale during the return movement. Use slow, deliberate motions instead than quick ones. For example, take 3 seconds to lift and exhale, 1 second to hold, and 3 seconds to lower and exhale. To improve tolerance, pause in between each repetition.

Resistance training can be done by participants two or more days a week, but they should avoid working out the same muscle area on consecutive days. Resistance training one day a week might be more beneficial and protective of the body than frequent exercise, and it's definitely lot more doable for people with FM.

It's crucial to warm up and cool down before and after any workout.

Remain persistent.

It's critical to maintain physical activity if you want to reap its benefits. Work your way up to a regular activity routine. It's likely that things will become better for you.

Ask your physical therapist or doctor for at-home workout recommendations if you need assistance getting started. When you're feeling well, take things slow so as not to overdo it. When you experience a flare-up of your fibro, dial it down. Locate a healthy equilibrium by paying attention to your body.

Psychological Therapies

- **Cognitive-Behavioral Therapy (CBT)**

Short-term psychological therapy known as cognitive behavioral therapy (CBT) is predicated on the idea that although our thoughts can impact our feelings and behaviors, our feelings and behaviors can also influence our thinking. Thus, we can learn to alter our feelings and behaviors by understanding how to alter the way we think.

Instead of being a single tactic, CBT is the general term for a collection of therapeutic approaches that are frequently combined. These approaches include journaling, mindfulness, acceptance and commitment therapy (ACT), which is a subtype of CBT that helps patients commit to acting in a way that is consistent with their values and accept their feelings as they are.

Cognitive behavioral therapy (CBT) is a goal-oriented, problem-solving therapeutic method that has been demonstrated to be beneficial for those with fibromyalgia in particular. It has also been shown to be effective for persons whose quality of life is negatively impacted by a chronic illness.

How ACT and CBT Can Benefit Fibromyalgia Patients

In a study that was published in the European Journal of Pain in April 2013, the researchers discovered that ACT improved the quality of life associated with mental health, pain-related functioning, self-efficacy, sadness, and anxiety in 40 fibromyalgia-affected women. Twelve weekly group ACT sessions were attended by the participants.

According to a research that was initially published in October 2011 in Arthritis Research & Therapy, CBT can aid fibromyalgia patients with pain catastrophizing. Generally speaking, catastrophizing is the belief that something is or will be far worse than it actually is. When someone engages in pain catastrophizing, he or she exaggerates the suffering they are actually or will experience.

Additional research has demonstrated that CBT can lessen fatigue, anxiety, and depression while enhancing sleep and day-to-day functioning. Furthermore, studies suggest that CBT, and specifically ACT, may be useful in minimizing feelings and experiences that exacerbate symptoms like stress and a loss of control, as well as in lessening the primary symptoms of fibromyalgia, which include pain, exhaustion, and fog in the brain.

CBT can help you manage some of the symptoms of fibromyalgia, according to Beth Kane, a licensed clinical social worker and life coach in Point Pleasant, New Jersey, who frequently works with patients with chronic illnesses.

☐ CBT Techniques for Handling Cognitive(Brain) Fog

"The weariness, chronic pain, and lack of restorative sleep a fibromyalgia patient may experience are thought to be attributed to brain fog," explains Kane. She claims that by utilizing CBT, which includes ACT, therapists may assist their patients in developing focused coping mechanisms and in making the required adjustments to more effectively handle upsetting situations.

One of these tactics is mindfulness, which is a part of ACT and is increasingly frequently employed in conjunction with CBT. "We are present-centered when we practice mindfulness. at that sense, we can more firmly access our consciousness at this exact instant, right here, right now, by using all five of our senses or bringing our awareness fully to the present moment, says Kane, rather than thinking or worrying about tomorrow or a month from now. You may be totally present in what you're doing when you practice mindfulness as opposed to getting mired in your thoughts.

She notes that visual processing and jotting down feelings or experiences in a notebook activates multiple brain regions and enables you to take a tangible action. Journaling is another technique she utilizes with her clients to help them focus.

☐ Overcoming Fatigue Applying CBT

There are several ways that CBT can assist with weariness.

"We can help clients identify tasks that are high-priority, recurring, or require high energy by using worksheets and journals. We can then plan a schedule around that, teaching them how to best utilize their time and energy."

By reducing the tension that can lead to weariness, the therapy can help the client manage these kinds of responsibilities.

"Helping them learn and use skills such as relaxation, acceptance, and mindfulness, and to recognize what they may be able to let go of in order to make better use of their energy," according to Kane, is another method that therapists can use CBT to combat fatigue.

☐ Changing the Way We Think About Pain

Another symptom that CBT addresses is pain. According to Kane, the purpose of the therapy is "to help reframe the thoughts about the pain, so that it doesn't become as consuming."

She gives the following example: "When thinking about pain, one might think, 'This pain is terrible and will never go away.'" A more accurate way to phrase it would be something like this: "This pain is terrible right now, but it will get better soon." I'll feel better soon, and I can get through this.

Alternatively, you can believe that "I can't live my life because of this pain."Rephrased, such idea might be, "I can still do x-y-z even though I'm in pain."

If you are in chronic pain, you are aware of how exhausting and wearing it can be. According to Kane, ACT can assist you in learning to accept your experiences as they are, which reduces expectation and deflects some of your attention from the discomfort.

☐ Reducing the Sensation of Being Out of Control

It can be frightening and frustrating for those suffering from chronic illnesses to feel as though they have no control over their body.

In an attempt to regain control, we may "get caught up in the 'what if' scenario or become so focused on our limitations that we can actually begin to insert even more limitations," according to Kane. This can exacerbate symptoms and increase anxiety and depressive symptoms.

"ACT also may be empowering, helping you question and see more clearly your own story, challenge any limiting beliefs, and learn to accept things as they really are, rather than how you imagine them to be," in addition to assisting you in accepting where you are at any given time.

☐ Using CBT to Learn How to Avoid Catastrophizing

The experience of suffering and a sense of being powerless that comes with having a chronic illness can both lead to catastrophizing, or what Kane refers to as "all-or-nothing, worst-possible-case-scenario thinking."

Once more, she cites the following as an illustration of a highly depressing thought: "This pain is stopping me from living my life." She claims that although you may have experienced periods of minimal pain and still managed to complete some tasks, it is sometimes simple to slip into these kinds of thought patterns.

According to her, you can use ACT to reframe the idea by asking yourself two questions:

Is that all true?

Does that idea support you in leading the life you desire?

Asking what is true and what would be helpful is important, she adds, if the answer to either or both of those questions is no. "Those responses can aid in reframing that disastrous idea."

☐ How to Locate a CBT Therapist

Find a therapist that can meet your unique needs and has experience working with individuals who have chronic illnesses if you'd want to investigate cognitive behavioral therapy. Get a recommendation from your physician for a licensed therapist.

• Mindfulness-Based Stress Reduction (MBSR)

An 8-week program called mindfulness-based stress reduction (MBSR) teaches mindfulness practices like yoga and meditation. Doctors may suggest it as a supplemental therapy in addition to other forms of care.

When the program first launched, it included: Weekly instructor-led group meditation sessions daily home guided meditation practice
 A full day mindfulness retreat in the sixth week
MBSR was first developed by Professor Jon Kabat-Zinn to help patients with chronic pain. Today's educators, however, have modified it for a variety of uses.

Encouraging people to concentrate their attention on the present moment is the main objective of MBSR. It entails concentrating on the body, embracing it, and letting go of the need to criticize, comprehend, or exert control.

Reducing stress has several health advantages, and practicing acceptance can help with that. In times of danger, humans can benefit from temporary stress. Chronic or long-term stress, however, is detrimental to numerous elements of health, including the immune system and sleep. By lowering the stress response, MBSR seeks to bring the body and mind back to a more relaxed condition.

☐ Examples and types

A variety of exercises can be included in MSBR;

Breathing:

This could involve a variety of breathing exercises. For instance, diaphragmatic breathing, sometimes referred to as belly breathing, can assist in lowering blood pressure and slowing the heartbeat.

Meditation:

There are numerous methods for doing this. In MBSR, body scan meditation is frequently used. This is paying attention to various body parts and letting go of each one. There's walking meditation, loving-kindness meditation, and more for those who find body scan meditations uncomfortable.

Yoga:

Yoga is a physical and mental discipline that has practitioners adjusting their poses while synchronizing their breathing.

Group discussion: In this, members of an MBSR group share their experiences. People talk about how they have incorporated MBSR into their regular routines during this exercise.

MBSR draws heavily from Eastern traditions, including Buddhism, for many of its concepts. But the main focus of MBSR is on the secular components of practices like yoga and meditation.

- Advantages of MBSR

MBSR can be used to treat or lessen the symptoms of a number of illnesses, such as:

An analysis of pain in 2019 According to a source of research, MBSR helped patients with lower back pain experience less pain-related distress, less severe pain, and fewer functional restrictions. The duration of these advantages was at least 52 weeks. Catastrophizing—assuming the worst—about pain is something that mindfulness may help prevent.

Stress: A Systematic Review from 2018 According to a prior research source, MBSR may assist in lowering employees' levels of stress and emotional tiredness. Emotional tiredness is a component of burnout, which is a significant health concern among workers.

The evaluation also identified significant improvements in sleep quality and self-compassion in study participants. The authors do point out that not all of the research they looked at were of a high caliber.

Depression and anxiety

Anxious or depressed persons can benefit from mindfulness. It functions by encouraging people to stay in the here and now rather than dwelling on the past or the future. In order to reach acceptance, MBSR can also assist with the processing of challenging emotions and experiences.

The advantages of MBSR might lessen how severe sadness and anxiety are. In a previous 2015 study, Trusted Source discovered that MBSR was just as successful at preventing relapses in depression as medications. Still, more investigation is required.

☐ Existing unintended consequences

The National Health Service (NHS) states that adverse effects with MBSR are uncommon. However, when engaging in mindfulness exercises like meditation, people could come across unprocessed feelings and thoughts.

Requiring one to slow down, mindfulness might cause feelings that one has not completely acknowledged to surface. Though it could get better with time, this can be challenging at first. It could be helpful to talk to one's instructor if mindfulness feels too intense or if it does not improve.

A person should think about calling a doctor if they encounter any other worrisome symptoms. The physician can confirm that these symptoms are not being caused by any underlying medical issues.

☐ How to use MBSR

Following an instructor-led, structured program is a requirement of MBSR. People can still practice mindfulness at home, though. An illustration of a body scan meditation is shown below.

☐ Meditation with a body scan

This practice involves focusing on the bodily feelings that an individual feels. To give it a shot:

1. Find a comfortable position to sit or lie in.
2. As soon as the body begins to relax, take several deep breaths in and out. If one so chooses, they can close their eyes.

3. Pay attention to how the feet feel, starting with the soles. Without passing judgment on them, pay attention to any feelings, whether they are good or bad.

4. Proceed progressively from the feet to the ankles and finally the legs, taking note of each area's unique sensation. One may want to deliberately tighten and loosen every muscle as they proceed.

5. Try to catch any instances where your focus stray from the body scan and gently bring it back.

6. A person can become aware of their entire body's sensations once they have reached their head. They have as much time as they want to remain in this meditative condition.

7. Open the eyes when you're ready.

MBR, or mindfulness-based stress reduction, is an adjunctive treatment. It can ease the symptoms of chronic pain, anxiety, and depression, and lower stress levels. MSBR focuses on teaching mindfulness practices that incorporate yoga or stretching, meditation, and breathing exercises.

At first, MBSR could be challenging. Broadly speaking, mindfulness can highlight unpleasant symptoms or emotions. On the other hand, staying in the moment can get easier with time.

It might be possible for those who are interested in MBSR to locate a local instructor. As an alternative, individuals can get advice from their physician.

• **Relaxation Techniques**

For those with FM, learning a relaxation method is a really helpful tool. Pain can be mitigated by relaxing your body; the more tight you are, the greater the pain will get. Learning to "push" your worries aside can help you cope with stress, worry, and depression. A peaceful mind can also help you think more clearly, rationalize your ideas, or just unwind for a bit.

There are "quick fix" relaxation methods that you can practice while seated at your desk for a few minutes during your hectic workday. These are not long-term solutions; rather, they provide a quick, harsh shock to the system, which is not what you need for chronic issues like FM.

For those suffering from FM The most effective methods are gradual, slow relaxations that affect your mental and physical health. You may learn to change your mental state at any time, so if you find yourself becoming worried about your discomfort, sense a panic attack coming on, or see that your mood is starting to deteriorate, you can take a break and distance yourself from everything.

As I previously stated, these aren't magic bullets; they require time and work. You must practice them whenever you can, if not every day. Consider that your homework for FM. While some people will find it easier than others, the benefits always outweigh the time and effort required, and the more you practice, the easier it will become. If it helps, picture a quiet, soothing voice guiding you.

Finding a place to unwind is the first step; different people have different needs in this regard. As long as you're comfortable and won't be disturbed, you can curl up in a beanbag, lie on the bed, or sit in your favorite chair.

After that, shut your eyes and focus on your breathing. Breathe more deeply and slowly as you take longer, more deliberate breaths. Take your time;

if you hurry, you won't have enough oxygen to do the task, and you'll be gasping and panting, which will negate the purpose.

When you are breathing deeply and slowly, picture yourself as though a warm, bright light is shining on you or that a part of your body is heavy. Next, pay close attention to that feeling and see it enveloping your entire being.

When you first try this, it usually helps to repeat this section a few times to help cement the experience. Alternatively, you can see the effect being stronger, heavier, warmer with each repetition. As a focus enhancer, counting up or down can be beneficial when performing this task.

The next step is to count to yourself while you visualize yourself descending, a little bit each count.

Remind yourself that you are gently and slowly descending, akin to a feather floating on the breeze. You've found your safe haven when you feel like you've hit rock bottom. Once more, this is a personal experience. It could be a real location, like your childhood bedroom, or it could be an imagined location, like a pleasant beach or meadow, where you feel safe and cherished. Take your time, visualize it completely, taking in all the colors, scents, and noises. Do birdsongs exist? Is there a scent of brewing coffee or wild flowers? For those of you who own pets, you may imagine them being a reassuring presence at your side. It's possible that there are some amiable creatures around, such as squirrels in the trees, bunnies playing on the grass, or birds perched on a tree branch outside a window. It's a bright, sunny, and breezy place, yet there's nothing chilly, frightful, or unsettling about it; everything is peaceful and pain- and stress-free.

You can think of positive affirmations and positive aspects of yourself when you are in your safe space. Statements beginning with "I," such as "I am strong," "I can do whatever," or "I will be able to do whatever," Simplify the statements as much as you can. You are more likely to leave your safe spot and try to recall them if they are more sophisticated because they will be tougher to remember. You can jot them down and keep them in front of you if you'd like. With experience, you'll be able to open your eyes and take a quick peek at them if necessary. Jot down the things that matter to you, the ways in which you wish to alter your perspective or your approach to things. If you are feeling low, write down statements like "I will feel happier today." If you are anxious, put down statements like "I will soon be able to go shopping on my own" or whatever your concern is.

If you're not worried about anything right now, simply stop by for a little bit, relax in the quiet, and take advantage of the opportunity to rest and adjust your pace. When you're done and feel prepared to return to reality, go SLOWLY. Instead of jumping up right soon, open your eyes gradually and take in your surroundings. Instead of getting out of bed or your chair right away, carefully extend your arms and legs as if you had been sleeping.

Once you can do this, you will always have your safe spot with you. To calm yourself down when you're feeling worried or upset, close your eyes for a while and visualize returning to your happy place. Allow the feelings that come with it to sweep over you. Just as "bad" feelings come over you when you think about something you don't like, all the feelings you have in your safe spot will come to you when you think about it.

As a note of caution, if you do this when you are out and about, make sure you are safe. It goes without saying that it is not a good idea to close your eyes while driving or crossing the street. Make sure no one is in your way as you pull over to the side of the road and pick a bench to relax on.

CHAPTER FOUR

ALTERNATIVE AND COMPLEMENTARY TREATMENTS

Acupuncture

Based on the idea that energy channels run beneath the skin's surface throughout the body, traditional Chinese medicine offers a therapeutic approach. These "meridians," or passageways, deliver essential materials to each and every cell, organ, tissue, bone, and joint in the human body.

The channels supply "homeostasis," or the ideal balance of fluids, temperature, and hormones, to every region of the body in addition to delivering blood, fluid, and a form of electrical energy, or "chi," to keep its systems operating.

The body consists of 14 main vessels that split into smaller channels to build a comprehensive network that nourishes different parts of our physical environment. The Chinese learned thousands of years ago that chi energy is concentrated at particular spots along the meridians. Additionally, they discovered that applying pressure to certain sites might affect the body's balance and health; this hypothesis gave rise to the creation of acupressure and acupuncture therapy. At these locations, an acupuncturist inserts tiny, specialized needles—tinier than a hair strand—into the skin. Modifying the flow of chi and "vital substances" (blood, lymph, and other bodily fluid circulation) in the afflicted meridians is the aim of treatment.

Every one of the 14 major vessels begins or finishes in one of the major organ systems. All the organs related to a meridian will be well supplied and work as intended as long as the flow of vital chemicals and chi remains unhindered.

Chinese medicine bases the preservation of the body's equilibrium and general health on two straightforward ideas:

1. The body needs enough chi and essential elements in the bloodstream to function correctly.

2. Illness arises when there is a deficiency or obstruction in the movement of chi and essential nutrients to the organs. A number of factors, such as

a poor diet, inefficient absorption and assimilation, an imbalance in the body's energy intake and production, or chronic illnesses that sap vitality, can cause this.

1. The inability of the body's systems to generate new energy, heal, and rebalance itself is exacerbated by a shortage of critical chemicals and chi.

Weakness, numbness, or coldness along the meridian itself, combined with failure of the organ system that the meridian is related to, are common signs of deficit in a meridian.

2. When one or more of the vessels are blocked, obstruction takes place.

In this instance, the mechanism is comparable to tossing a log into a stream. There will be a shortfall downstream, past the obstacle, and a backlog in one region if the flow of chi is blocked. The backlog and deficit it creates increase with the length of time the meridian is blocked. A number of things can cause obstruction, such as physical trauma (which results in swelling and bruises that obstruct the passage of chi) and stress and tension (which causes the meridians to constrict and restrict the flow of chi). When a meridian is blocked, it can cause discomfort, heat, or weight along the meridian, as well as problems with the organ system that the meridian is attached to.

☐ Diagnosis

Finding out which meridians are blocked or inadequate and why is the main goal of diagnosis in traditional Chinese medicine. The meridian system is interrelated, therefore indications of deficiency or obstruction, like pain or numbness in a meridian, may originate in a completely different area of the body. Just treating the location where the pain or numbness is present would be a simple solution. But when the problem's core causes are properly recognized and dealt with, the course of treatment is much more efficient and long-lasting.

A crucial component of any acupuncture treatment is diagnosis. Finding the true root cause(s) of the patient's ailment may take some time for the acupuncturist, depending on how severe and chronic the problem is. Because of this, an acupuncturist's initial diagnostic session may last an hour or longer, and the diagnosis is continuously reviewed during all subsequent therapy sessions.

Treatment aims to restore the flow of vital substances and chi in the damaged organs and meridians once the imbalances have been discovered. Stimulating points that are known to affect the appropriate places help to rebalance chi. Chinese herbal medicine and acupuncture are frequently combined. In addition, heat therapy, massage, and dietary or exercise advice may be part of the treatment.

☐ Acupuncture For FM

FM is diagnosed under three different categories in traditional Chinese medicine.
There are components of deficit and blockage in every diagnosis:

1. Heat trapping

This pertains particularly to the disequilibrium that arises from an invasive bacterial or viral infection that remains unresolved within the body.

When a patient's defenses are weakened by stress or sleep deprivation, this can happen. The body's defense mechanism may be further weakened if the infection is not eliminated. In this instance, the outcome is frequently a form of trapped heat (inflammation) that gets worse anytime the patient feels fatigued or under a lot of stress. In this situation, pain is frequently searing in character. Additional concomitant symptoms include fever (particularly at night), mouth sores, sore throats, scorching skin, sleeplessness, restlessness, exhaustion, and irritability. The goal of treatment is to restore the flow of vital substances and chi in the afflicted meridians while also cooling the body by applying spots that specifically eliminate heat.

2. Moistness or moisture combining with heat

Natural metaphors are used in traditional Chinese medicine to explain bodily ailments. Conditions known as dampness in FM manifest as a build-up of fluid, mucus discharge, swelling, or edema that obstructs the organs and meridians. An imbalance in the kidney or digestive systems of the body may be the cause of this. A diet overly high in sugary foods and things that make the body retain fluid and generate phlegm may also be to blame. This pattern of symptoms frequently includes feelings of heaviness, numbness, and swelling in addition to pain. Additional symptoms may include weight gain, lethargy, insomnia, depression, low appetite, loose stools, nausea, swollen glands, and headaches. The discomfort will be both heavy and scorching if the moist state combines with heat that is trapped in the body. Toxicological indicators may also include the following symptoms: greasy hair and skin with recurrent skin eruptions, strong bodily odors, agitation, and extreme sleeplessness.

3. Inadequate chi and essential elements

In these situations, the body's vital vitality has gradually decreased in the past. This could be the outcome of a protracted illness, a traumatic event involving a significant blood loss, a persistently bad diet, burning the candle at both ends, or an excessively depleted workout habit.

Malnutrition impairs the body's meridians and organs, making it harder for the body to maintain healthy circulation and keep substances flowing through the meridians, which leads to obstruction and further deterioration in health.

In many instances, the pain is dull in nature and gets worse with movement. Poor circulation, pale skin, a propensity to feel chilly or numb, palpitations, exhaustion, dyspnea, dizziness, or unsteadiness in balance are some other symptoms that may be present.

In conclusion, acupuncture treatments can be quite useful in reducing symptoms if a patient exhibits any of the above listed symptoms. A deficiency happens when the body does not have enough chi or other essential components.

Massage Therapy

It's amazing how many advantages massage can offer those with FM . I strongly advise you to see a massage therapist with experience treating FM if you have had a negative experience with massage treatment.

When performed properly, massage can be highly beneficial, but it can also be quite unpleasant if you visit the incorrect individual. I believe your condition will improve significantly if you can locate a massage therapist with experience treating illnesses similar to yours.

Typically, I start by hearing the history of a new patient. I frequently try to address the significant emotional component that a FM patient has because they have been experiencing both physical and emotional discomfort. They come to me disillusioned and often melancholy, having seen very little progress by the time they come. They are frequently frustrated. I understand their predicament because, in addition to their symptoms, they are going through the stress response, which is the sympathetic nervous system's response to the discomfort and stressful circumstances they are going through. They are extremely "bound up" in their bodies, have tight muscles, and typically breathe shallowly. Numerous holding patterns and guarding behaviors are present.

The massage therapist must establish a safe space before they can begin working with patients. The intention is to assist patients feel less anxious and more empathic toward them. Without really offering counseling, I make an effort to emotionally connect with my patients. Many of my patients are attempting to address their emotional problems and also see mental health counselors.

Ensuring a secure atmosphere is crucial, particularly during the initial phases of treatment, to enable the patient to make decisions about their likeness and comfort level with you. If they feel uncomfortable and the practitioner is only working on their tense, rigid muscles, there's a good chance they will relax more and respond to treatment more effectively in a safe and comfortable setting. To help the patient unwind, I like to make the massage room somewhat warm. There's quiet music playing, low lighting, and a hint of aromatherapy in the air. This makes it possible for the sufferer to unwind both physically and mentally.

The initial meeting is crucial for evaluating the patient and gauging their current state of disease. When it comes to treating someone who has just received a FM diagnosis, I am extremely cautious and conservative.

A common request from patients who have recently received an FM diagnosis is for me to go very deeply into the painful portions of their bodies. I have to explain to them how massage affects their body because, although the manipulation may feel good during the session, the areas that have been worked on may be so painful the following day that you've actually done more harm than good. Tapping those specific points can actually cause a much more severe flare-up the following day. For this reason, it's critical to start treating patients with FM with extreme caution.

Working with individuals who have FM and CFS is incredibly fascinating. It's difficult because there isn't any predetermined foundation and you need to have a wide range of talents in order to assist everyone. While a patient with a muscle strain or sprain would often receive the same care each time they see you, you wouldn't always treat a FM patient the same way.

Giving patients the chance to reflect and get grounded for themselves is a big part of what I do; their own healing process will take care of the issues they have been whining about. It's far more difficult to move forward when one is caught in a loop of resistance; it's like bumping against people instead of flowing with the situation.

Although massage is beneficial, one shouldn't expect it to heal anything. When used in conjunction with other therapies, it can be highly helpful and help you progress more quickly because it promotes personal healing. It can help you feel better every day and get you back on the path to recovery much more quickly.

Chiropractic Care

Many people are unaware that chiropractors are medical professionals. Chiropractors attend a four-year chiropractic college, much like medical doctors attend a four-year medical school. During the first two years, the programs are quite similar, with most courses addressing basic sciences, microbiology, cell biology, biochemistry, and anatomy and physiology. The final two years of graduate school are where chiropractic and medical schools diverge.

Students at chiropractic colleges learn how to use soft tissue therapy, exercise, diet, physical therapy, and spinal adjustments to promote the body's natural healing processes. The medical method involves employing medicine or surgery to address the symptom or issue.

Chiropractors are accepted as primary care physicians in the United States. After diagnosing a wide range of illnesses, we either treat the patient or recommend them to the proper medical facility. Neuromusculoskeletal (NMS) diseases are a specialty of chiropractors. The skeletal, muscular, and neurological systems are all impacted by these NMS disorders.

Of this kind, FM and CFS are two that chiropractors treat with remarkable success.

A chiropractor specializes in the diagnosis and treatment of spinal subluxations, which are misaligned or asymmetrically movable vertebrae that impair normal nervous system function. Pain and dysfunction can result from misaligned or constricted spine because these conditions negatively impact the nerves and muscles. Your brain and the rest of your body are constantly in communication thanks to your nerve system. The nerve system's pressure or tension prevents the brain and body from communicating normally. Pressure on the neurological system may be the cause of the chronic pain patterns observed in FM and CFS patients.

Prior to beginning any patient's treatment, a comprehensive examination enables the chiropractor to identify any vertebral subluxation and makes the dysfunctional area known to the patient. To identify the locations of vertebral subluxation, a comprehensive examination includes postural assessment, palpation (moving the spine and muscles gently), orthopedic testing, and chiropractic tests. X-rays are frequently used to identify structural misalignments and to rule out other potential diseases or underlying issues.

A typical chiropractic examination involves a lot of hands-on work. The chiropractor must measure the vertebrae and spine's range of motion to ascertain which parts can move freely and which feel constrained. Additionally, the muscles must be examined to identify any abnormal tension or spasms. The examination for FM and CFS patients will differ depending on the level of pressure that may be applied, particularly when palpating.

A relative measure of sensitivity is necessary since the muscles and tissues are hypersensitive.

The spinal adjustment is the main therapeutic technique used by chiropractors.

The hands-on kind of modification is the most popular. When a section of the spine is misaligned, the chiropractor uses appropriate force—which can range from very light to firm—with his or her hands to realign the spine and enhance function. The nervous system is relieved and the body starts to mend normally when the vertebrae are repositioned and have their natural range of motion. Numerous adjusting instruments can also be used to deliver an adjustment. Improving the nervous system's and spine's function is the aim of every correction.

There are numerous variations in chiropractic methods. Some people's main worry is whether the adjustment will hurt, although most chiropractic adjustments don't. Those who were worried frequently say something like, "That felt great," or even, "That wasn't bad." Tell your chiropractor about any worries you may have; a skilled chiropractor will use adjustment methods that both help you feel better and produce desired outcomes. Effective communication can also assist allay any additional worries you may have.

A skilled chiropractor will use adjustment methods that both feel natural to you and produce desired outcomes. Effective communication can also assist allay any additional worries you may have.

Dietary Supplements

- 5-Hydroxytryptophan, or 5-HTP

This dietary supplement is a precursor to serotonin. Serotonin is a potent neurotransmitter, and fibromyalgia pain is significantly influenced by serotonin levels. Sleep and depression are also linked to serotonin levels.

5-HTP can help both men and women with fibromyalgia sleep deeper and experience less discomfort. In a study done in 2015, researchers found that taking 5-HTP supplements could help with fibromyalgia pain, anxiety, sleeplessness, and depression symptoms. Contradictory research, however, indicate that 5-HTP has no beneficial effects.

5-HTP is often well accepted. However, the supplement was linked to the dangerous eosinophilia-myalgia syndrome in the late 1980s. The illness, which manifests as flu-like symptoms, excruciating muscle pain, and searing rashes, is believed to have been caused by a contamination in 5-HTP.

☐ Melatonin

A supplement containing this hormone can be purchased over-the-counter. It can occasionally be used to enhance sleep patterns and cause drowsiness. Melatonin may be useful in the treatment of fibromyalgia pain, according to some early research. It is believed that melatonin may help alleviate the exhaustion, muscle soreness, and sleep issues that the majority of fibromyalgia sufferers experience. Most people agree that melatonin is safe and has few to no negative effects. Until they are familiar with how melatonin affects them, people using it should exercise caution when driving due to the possibility of daytime sleepiness.

- John's Wort

Although St. John's wort is frequently used to treat depression, which is frequently linked to fibromyalgia, there is no concrete proof that it is beneficial in treating fibromyalgia.

In the short run, St. John's wort is as effective as earlier antidepressants known as tricyclics and more effective than a placebo in treating mild to moderate depression, according to several studies. According to other research, St. John's wort is just as successful in treating depression as certain SSRI antidepressants like Zoloft or Prozac.

St. John's wort is generally not harmful. Fatigue, skin responses, and unsettled stomachs are the most frequent adverse effects. Antidepressants and St. John's wort shouldn't be combined because it can interact with a variety of medications.

Tell a doctor if you take medication before taking any supplements, including St. John's wort. Additionally, use caution while using St. John's wort with other medications, such as antidepressants.

☐ SAM-e

The exact mechanism of action of SAM-e in the body is unknown. Some people believe that this natural substance raises dopamine and serotonin levels, two neurotransmitters in the brain.

Current trials do not appear to indicate any effect of SAM-e over placebo in reducing the number of tender points or treating depression associated with fibromyalgia, despite the belief held by some researchers that SAM-e may change mood and promote restful sleep. Further research is required to validate these results. According to the University of Maryland Medical Center, the suggested dosage for fibro research is 400 mg twice day for six weeks. To prevent stomach disturbance, the amount should be progressively increased from a beginning point of roughly 200 mg daily. But ask your doctor; each patient has a different dosage.

- L-aspartate

Despite the paucity of research, L-carnitine is believed to alleviate pain and address additional fibromyalgia symptoms. Researchers assessed the efficacy of L-carnitine in 102 fibromyalgia patients in a single small trial.

The L-carnitine group significantly improved their symptoms compared to the placebo-taking control group, according to the results. The researchers came to the conclusion that, although further research is necessary, L-carnitine may help fibromyalgia sufferers with their pain and enhance their overall and mental health.

☐ Magnesium

One of the vitamins and nutritional supplements required for strong, healthy muscles and brains is magnesium. Regardless of the existence of any pain issues, the Food and Drug Administration recommends that persons 19 years of age and older consume 400–420 mg of magnesium per day for males and 310–320 mg per day for women. The majority of your daily magnesium needs should be met by diet, and you should always get medical advice before incorporating vitamin supplements into your diet.

Low magnesium levels can exacerbate the symptoms of illnesses including chronic pain. A 2021 study discovered a connection between magnesium deficit and typical fibromyalgia symptoms like anxiety, insomnia, weariness, and muscular soreness.

- Vitamin D

The benefits of the "sunshine vitamin" extend beyond bone growth.

It can also aid in the fight against fatigue and fibro pain, per a 2014 study that was published in the journal Pain.

Thirty women with fibromyalgia, who also lacked vitamin D, were split into two groups for the study. For 20 weeks, the therapy group took oral vitamin

D supplements. The group under control was given a placebo.

Within a week, the group receiving therapy experienced a significant decrease in pain, reduced morning weariness than the placebo group, and better physical functioning.

Our best source of vitamin D is sun exposure, which causes the skin to create it. However, the National Institutes of Health state that some people don't make enough of the vitamin. These include obese, dark-skinned, and older ladies.

Individuals who suffer from specific conditions, such as Crohn's or celiac disease, or who wear sunscreen or don't get enough sunshine are also susceptible to deficiencies.

The simplest approach to make sure you get enough vitamin D is to consume pills, as few foods contain it.

The National Institutes of Health state that the recommended daily intake of vitamin D is 600 international units (IU) for individuals aged 1 to 70 and 800 IU for those aged 71 and above, with a daily maximum of 4,000 IU.

However, find out from your physician how much you should take to manage your fibro symptoms.

☐ Fish Oil

Fish oil has excellent anti-inflammatory qualities because of its omega-3 fatty acids, which can help lessen fibro discomfort.

It lessens the body's synthesis of prostaglandins, which are inflammatory hormones, according to board-certified rheumatologist Nehad Soloman, M.D. of Valley Arthritis Care in Arizona. And less stiffness or sore joints could result from that.

While fish oil supplements are thought to be safe, Dr. Soloman advises selecting a brand that is mercury-free (read the label).

To lower inflammation and strengthen your immune system, take one or two capsules (or one or two teaspoons) per day, suggests the University of Maryland Medical Center. However, see your physician first, particularly if you use any blood thinners like aspirin or warfarin (Coumadin).

☐ Ribose

Fibro discomfort is frequently caused by tense muscles. Muscles require energy to release and relax. And ribose pills are useful in this situation.

According to a 2012 study, ribose, a simple sugar, can reduce fibromyalgia sufferers' pain by an average of 15.6% and improve energy by an average of 61%.

According to the study, "the energy-building benefit of ribose directly improved the debilitating symptoms of this condition."

A 5g dosage three times a day is advised.

☐ Extract from Brown Seaweed

These pills might be unfamiliar to you, but this is a supplement worth looking into.

According to Dr. Soloman, "it's showing great promise in the fight against chronic pain."

In fact, a 2011 study from Australia's Centre of Health and Wellbeing published in the journal Biologics found that ingesting 1,000 mg of brown seaweed extract daily can reduce joint pain and stiffness by 52%.

Even better: You won't have to wait long to find out if it works for you because these benefits started to show results after just one week.

You should inquire of your doctor the following:

1. What is the appropriate dosage for me?
2. Should I eat before taking it?
3. When should I take it during the day?
4. Will my prescription drugs and this supplement interact negatively?
5. Does it have any adverse effects that could resemble or worsen my fibro symptoms, including depression or trouble sleeping?

Herbal remedies and flower essence

I fell in love with our land the day we moved to Tree Frog Farm. To get better at listening, I would stroll around and let the plants talk to me and draw me in. I gained knowledge about planting and maintaining gardens, cleansing land of energy, and taking care of the woods in harmony with the environment. I started creating my own flower essences there.

Those with FM, in my experience, are naturally sensitive individuals. Many are stuck in the "fight or flight" mode of stress, which leads to hypersensitivity to almost everything. In these situations, the first essential oils I employ support a decrease in hypersensitivity and trauma from the body-mind-spirit continuum. I frequently utilize bleeding heart, moon shadow rose, lady's mantle, pennyroyal, and comfrey in similar circumstances. I occasionally also use purple passion rose, self-heal, and imitation orange.

Pennyroyal; Calms the sympathetic nervous system. From a spiritual perspective, it gives you courage to maintain your center of gravity and then let go when the apparent threat passes. (This mostly addresses a survival issue with the kidney system and adrenal gland.)

Lady's Mantle: By regulating the sympathetic nervous system, it offers profound spiritual serenity to your entire body and essence. (This primarily deals with emotional heart shock, which triggers the sympathetic nervous system.)

Comfrey: Helps repair traumatizing and deeply ingrained wounds that interfere with the soul's journey.

Bleeding Heart: Encourages self-compassion in difficult or stressful circumstances. helps in the transition from wanting to alter other people or circumstances to realizing that the only things you can change are yourself and how you respond to them.

Moon Shadow Rose: Invites us to let go of the ghosts of the past and be receptive to the lessons they can teach us.

Mock Orange: Cleanses your cells and extracts emotional residue.

Self-Heal: By balancing the chakras down the spine, this technique helps to promote the condition of equilibrium from which entire body/being integration flows.

The purple passion rose helps to break through entangled karmic patterns.

My customers primarily take the floral essences orally—one drop in a glass of water or in their mouths. On occasion, I apply a drop of self-heal flower essence, pennyroyal, or comfrey flower essence to a client's sore spots near the base of their skull using my fingertips. Lady's mantle and bleeding heart are beneficial for spots on the front of the neck and upper chest.

Flower essences are a simple self-care tool for everybody. However, patients with FM frequently are limited to taking one drop daily, or perhaps one every other day, and at first are only allowed to use three essences at a time. The floral essence can be applied straight from the dropper onto your arms or torso points if you're lying down. Alternatively, dab the essence on your finger first, then gently touch the area that feels sore. Make sure the dropper doesn't come into contact with your skin or anything else. In that case, simply give the dropper a quick wash in warm water before putting it back in the container.

According to my philosophy, everyone of us is a spark of the creative life force, evolving through experiences to discover more about who we are. We often lose sight of our identity. Traumatic learning experiences have the potential to lodge in our bodies and cause physical problems. In order to learn and advance on their spiritual journeys, I advise my clients to remember who they are and to let go of old energetic holdings layer by layer. (This mostly addresses a survival issue with the kidney system and adrenal gland.)

MIND-BODY PRACTICES

• YOGA FOR FIBROMYALGIA SUFFERERS

Yoga is a type of Eastern exercise and movement therapy that helps the body regain its flexibility, balance, and functionality. The body should be in good health and the mind should be at ease, according to ancient philosophy. I started doing yoga when I was in my mid-forties. I felt really wonderful about it that I wasn't content to merely lounge around watching TV with my body. Although many people mistakenly believe that yoga is just for stretching, regular practice also strengthens and nourishes the body's internal organs and other systems. I also like the benefits of deep relaxation that come from quieting the body; the body's energies then flow into the immune system, which further supports the body's vitality.

When a student confided in me that she had FM and was 90% pain-free after taking my class, I became interested in FM. This inspired me to create a workshop specifically for individuals with FM. We work with the assumption that there is pain in this session, and our objective is to move and stretch without making the discomfort worse. The "Fibromyoga" class is kept as small as possible by myself. Every client has unique needs. Some clearly exhibit physical issues, while others do not. One is unable to rotate, and another has movement-inhibiting issues with their hips and knees. Everyone understands that their bodies are their own teachers and that they have the freedom to choose what is good for them and to disregard what is not. I once learned from a yoga instructor that if she enters a class and finds every student engaged in the same activity at the same moment, she can be certain that the teacher is incompetent and hasn't given the students the tools they need to become lifelong learners. In spite of my customized approach, my classes follow a set structure.

☐ A GENTLE CLASS

Students enter my workshop through a landscape with pools and flowing water designed in the Japanese manner. There are many of pillows and blankets in the carpeted studio. On chilly mornings, I construct a fire in the fireplace and warm stones for folks to hold in their hands. It is suggested that students enter the room, lie down, and unwind. If they'd want, they can use the stones to warm their bodies as well. At that moment, we all check in, sharing our feelings and disclosing any significant changes to our bodies since the previous lesson. Sometimes we chant "Om" at the start of class as a way to honor the long-standing yoga tradition. In addition to breathing exercises and eye movements, I also teach abdominal cleansing techniques that are meant to clear the digestive tract. The Sun Salutation is the next exercise we perform as a warm-up. The standing, twisting, forward-bending, and backward-bending poses are the basis of the lesson. I teach poses that are quite soft, and after moving for a little while, we rest in a stance known as restorative pose. The body can regenerate itself in the resting stances, where it exerts little to no effort. This method also fortifies the immune system when paired with deep relaxation and mild stretching. An exercise in profound relaxation concludes the program. We can hear natural sounds like rushing water when the windows are open during warm weather, so I occasionally play relaxing music in the background.

☐ LOCATING A YOGA EXPERT

A skilled yoga instructor must to possess a number of traits. They ought to get certified first. They ought to have studied under another instructor, ideally from a different lineage of yoga than their own. I teach a very gentle style of yoga, but there are many other lineages; some are really demanding. All of these traditions should be familiar to the yoga instructor.) A fundamental understanding of the body's anatomy and functions is essential for a yoga instructor. They ought to be able to identify the main muscles. Go for another teacher if you inquire where the biceps are and they reply, "In the legs." They ought to be able to identify the skeleton's principal bones as well. I instruct a moderate style of yoga called "integral yoga," in which most postures are done while sitting or lying down, interspersed with lots of rest intervals. You might need to stay away from other more strenuous types of yoga if you have FM. Iyengar yoga, for instance, requires a lot of standing poses and is highly taxing. "Bikram yoga" is done in an extremely hot atmosphere and is equally strenuous. Power yoga incorporates a continuous sequence of poses that flow from one to the next without pause, therefore it calls for more power and endurance.

Yoga helps us become totally present to our bodies, allowing us to become fully aware of their processes. For a few period, we are able to put the past and future behind us and focus on the present, when happiness and tranquility may be found. We might even temporarily forget about our physical discomforts. Spiritual awareness is piqued by this, but on a physical level, it just feels nice to move without experiencing pain—or as she puts it, "Go elsewhere in the legs." They ought to be able to identify the skeleton's principal bones as well.

Tai Chi and Qigong

Millions of people worldwide, including millions in China, practice the movement and meditation arts of tai chi and qigong, which have their roots in China. Qigong, which is the study of vital force, or "qi" (chi, spelled differently in Chinese), is one of the oldest disciplines.

Man was formed in the past for spiritual and physical well-being. Currently, it's estimated that there are over 10,000 distinct types of qigong, some of which have been practiced for over 2,000 years and some of which were created by qigong professionals recently. The five main groups of Qigong are medicinal, martial, Buddhist, Taoist, and confusion. It is a cornerstone of traditional Chinese medicine as a therapeutic modality and is prescribed for a wide range of medical conditions, including lowering blood pressure and stress, enhancing the immune and endocrine systems, and fortifying the cardiovascular system. It is also used in conjunction with acupuncture, massage, and herbs. Grand ultimate boxing, or tai chi ch'uan, has its origins in the early 1600s.

Although tai chi was originally developed primarily by a few prominent families as a self-defense technique, it is now primarily recognized as a type of focused exercise. It is regarded as a form of qigong, and qigong-like benefits are associated with it. Tai chi also helps with balance and general motor control, which is particularly beneficial for the lower limbs.

Although there are many variations in tai chi and qigong practices, all involve relaxation, calmness of mind and body, fluid movement, and coordinated diaphragmatic breathing. The exercises vary in pace from being quiet and contemplative to being busy and rather intense. In general, tai chi and qigong forms consist of a series of complimentary motions that are performed constantly and mostly slowly. The routines follow a rhythm where they progress from stillness to movement, with each action flowing naturally into the next, before coming to a conclusion with a return to rest. Both the body and the intellect are fully focused. Unlike other traditional activities that focus on the physical body through muscle strengthening or stretching, the primary goal of tai chi and qigong is to build and balance chi first.

Good news for people with FM: qigong and tai chi are types of exercise. These exercise techniques are essential for improving breathing, mental clarity, and relaxation. This technique improves blood flow, tissue repair, and organ function by releasing chi stagnation and obstructions. Since relaxation is the primary goal of tai chi and qigong, practicing these techniques also improves one's capacity to more effectively affect their own autonomic, sympathetic, and parasympathetic nervous systems. This translates into an easier time transitioning out of the stress reaction.

A practitioner of tai chi and qigong has numerous health benefits, much like a highly trained athlete. Studies from China and an increasing number of Western researches demonstrate the health benefits of meditation exercise, which include lowered blood pressure, improved cardiac fitness, bolstered immunological and musculoskeletal systems, improved balance and coordination, and an overall sense of well-being.

The student of tai chi and qigong achieves these goals without running the risk of injury from overstretching their bodies, in contrast to other more strenuous sports. When done correctly, tai chi and qigong do not result in muscle rips, spasms, or electrolyte loss. Furthermore, none of the exercises cause the body to release an excessive amount of adrenaline to be pushed through it, unlike weightlifting, which does. This is crucial for people with health issues like FM, as their bodies have trouble metabolizing adrenaline.

☐ A STORY OF SUCCESS

I was hired by a doctor at a nearby hospital in the middle of the 1990s to create a tai chi and qigong program for his patients who suffered from chronic pain. My mobility and exercise program was made to help patients function and get some pain relief so they wouldn't need to visit the pain clinic as frequently. The majority of participants in this program had severe health issues, such as FM and CFS, and were in excruciating agony. We together discovered how to combine movement with the principles of tai chi and qigong for fatigue syndromes and chronic pain.

Among the program's participants was Candace S., a landscaper and athlete in her early 50s. She had spent her entire life being slender, strong, and energetic. She had the illness about two years before she started the program, and she never fully recovered. Candace was nearly bedridden and fifty pounds overweight when she enrolled in the eight-week program. Candace had been misdiagnosed with FM for some time, having been a puzzle to the medical establishment.

Candace could not stand for longer than two minutes without her pulse rate rising beyond 200 beats per minute when she started taking my classes. Candace did her best to follow the routines for the entire eight weeks, taking a break every two minutes.

Candace would pay close attention throughout the rest period, ingraining the basic arm, waist, and leg movements into her memory. She would close her eyes and obey the verbal commands when watching got too taxing.

Candace got good at imagining the motions and would mentally rehearse them at home. We saw Candace start to stand and practice the exercises with the group for at least half of the class period after just four weeks of practice.

In this fashion, Candace continued honing her tai chi and qigong abilities, and over the course of the following four years, she began to practice for hours on end, many days a week.

She excelled academically and continued her education with other instructors to become a capable assistant instructor. Although Candace didn't completely eradicate her FM or rely solely on qigong and tai chi exercises to enhance her well-being, they played a significant role in reducing her symptoms and significantly raising her standard of living.

The ability to become more aware is arguably the best gift that practicing tai chi and qigong can give a learner who has FM. A pupil gains increased awareness of all of his or her motions—not just in practice but also in daily life—because the technique's deliberate, uninterrupted movements place a strong focus on conscious awareness. Through training, a learner learns to become more self-aware and adapt their form for better balance and fluidity. It is simple to apply this ability to life in general. Students studying FM can learn to identify common movement patterns that lead to pain and then modify them. Additionally, a student may learn to recognize and alter mental patterns that result in tense movements.

☐ IDENTIFYING A QIGONG OR TAI CHI TEACHER

Choosing the correct teaching setting and a qualified instructor is crucial when starting a tai chi or qigong practice. Even though these are age-old methods, they are still relatively new to the world of fitness in general and even more so when viewed as a form of therapy. To find the perfect fit, some research might be necessary. In particular, I have found that because tai chi requires more movement and less standing, it may be somewhat more beneficial for those with severe FM. Qigong is usually more beneficial for CFS sufferers since it requires less activity and may be easily adapted to sitting and sleeping positions.

It is usually preferable, though, to give yourself some time to figure out what suits you.

We do not recommend watching videos or DVDs to learn for those with FM. Although the designs appear straightforward, there is a unique structural and energy alignment. Self-correction is a challenging task for individuals, and doing the forms wrong might result in an injury, spasm, or flare-up.

☐ SEARCHING FOR THE IDEAL TEACHER

1. Pay more attention to the teacher's personality and heart than to their credentials. Finding a trained teacher is fantastic, but certification programs are not common. Look for a teacher that is understanding and prepared to hear your needs and limitations. The instructor should also be open to discussing how the form might be changed to better suit your needs.

2. Work with a teacher who has been teaching for a number of years. Your teacher should be highly attuned to energy and physical alignment, and have a refined, empathic teaching approach that comes from working with a wide range of students.

3. Look for a learning environment that suits your needs. You should be motivated to attend class if it is laid back, friendly, and noncompetitive. Remind your teacher, if needed, that scented items like incense and perfume should not be used in a

training setting. You should always have access to a cozy chair so you may sit and relax when needed.

☐ BEING AVAILABLE AS A TOP STUDENT:

1. Take the initiative to learn. Find out if filling out the form while sitting down. Request a break in between workouts. Your teacher will respond "yes" if they are good!

2. Proceed cautiously. Although qigong and tai chi are gentle, they can nevertheless be overused. Remain mindful, remain alert, and cease before you believe it is necessary. Small amounts have a big impact.

3. Exercise patience. Qigong and tai chi provide gradual, cumulative advantages. These are methods that are not frequently associated with the way we think about exercise and movement. Consider the

procedure first. Instead of seeing the exercise as a destination, let it become your path.

Qigong and tai chi are great for regaining equilibrium, reducing pain, and—most importantly—bringing back the joy of being a living human. I've found that patients with FM can benefit greatly from tai chi and qigong in terms of their health. They work best, though, when combined with additional techniques including acupuncture, physical therapy, dietary counseling, and emotional coaching. Whichever method you decide on, the main idea behind these exercises is to move slowly and deliberately while constantly aiming for relaxation. Make as many changes as necessary to suit your comfort level, and speak with your teacher personally. Like life, tai chi and qigong really work best when we learn to let go and let our natural fluidity come through.

CHAPTER FIVE

LIFESTYLE MODIFICATIONS AND SELF-CARE

Diet and Nutrition

It's not hard to eat the appropriate foods when you have fibro. You just need to adhere to a few fundamental guidelines and keep in mind a few things. Red meat is difficult to recall. Were you aware that green peppers include a substance known as solanine that modifies the way muscles' enzymes work, resulting in pain? Is ginger a potent antioxidant as well? We avoid heavy, starchy foods and avoid eating eggplant since we find them difficult to tolerate. Our diets are free of sugar, fat, and sodium. But fear not, fans of sweets—we can still enjoy naturally sweet foods like fruit and honey! Instead of using white flour, we use spelt flour. We adore soy butter and rice noodles. We dress our salads with flaxseed oil and extra virgin olive oil. Numerous options exist to fulfill every desire.

☐ Basic Dietary components in Fibromyalgia
Fatigue is one of the most prevalent signs and symptoms of fibromyalgia. Eating foods that offer you energy is one of the finest strategies to combat the tiredness you feel:

1. Dark leaves Greens. These consist of watercress, broccoli, collard greens, mustard greens, bok choi, arugula, and spinach.

2. Bananas. Bananas are among the fruits that will provide you with the greatest energy for your money. The fruit of choice for athletes competing in long-distance races. It contains high amount of potassium, vitamin B6, and is carbohydrate-rich.

3. Sweet potatoes. Sweet potatoes are a nutrient powerhouse in addition to being delicious. They also include manganese, a mineral that functions similarly to iron in the body and aids in converting dietary nutrients into even more energy.

4. Good fats. Nuts, avocados, fatty salmon, and extra virgin olive oil are some examples of these.

5. Protective agents. Antioxidant-rich foods shield nerve cells from touch sensitivity. Berries, kidney beans, artichokes, pecans, beets, spinach, and dark

chocolate are examples of these kinds of foods. Because dietary excitotoxins can cause oxidative stress, you may need to increase the amount of antioxidants in your diet to counteract their impact on fibromyalgia symptoms.

"To keep things simple, look for fruits and vegetables that add color to your diet". "To give oneself an antioxidant boost, concentrate on boosting consumption of items with vivid red, green, orange, yellow, and purple hues."

6. Omega-3s. Omega-3 fatty acid-rich foods have an anti-inflammatory impact, which is beneficial for aching joints. Salmon, Brussels sprouts, eggs, chia seeds, walnuts, sardines, flax seeds, and soybeans are among the foods in this group.

☐ Foods to Steer Clear of If You Have Fibromyalgia

Since symptoms might vary greatly from person to person, it is recommended that you maintain a food journal in order to monitor flare-ups. It will be simpler to pinpoint the precise food kinds that are actively aggravating your ailment in this approach.

1. Meats that are cured or crimson. Anything that has preservatives or salt added can make your body inflamed. Red meats are no different.

2. Artificial trans fats and fried meals. The following foods exacerbate fibromyalgia symptoms: french fries, onion rings, funnel cake, donuts, margarine, shortening, vegetable oils, and peanut oil.

3. Limit Sugar and Steer Clear of Artificial Sweeteners.

Holton advises staying away from artificial sweeteners including sucralose, aspartame, acesulfame-K, and saccharin. When sweetening meals, use honey or ordinary sugar minimally.

"If you aren't using artificial sweeteners, it's much easier to wean yourself off of sugar," she explains.

You'll be able to detect sweetness in meals more readily when you reduce your sugar intake. Since stevia is hundreds of times sweeter than sugar, you naturally want your meal to be sweeter.

Steer clear of high-fructose corn syrup for overall wellness. If you're feeling low on energy due to fibromyalgia, avoid using sugar or corn syrup substitutes. Consuming a lot of sugar raises the risk of diabetes, weight gain, and other inflammatory illnesses like cancer and heart disease.

According to research, the body needs a lot of energy to cope with excitotoxicity, says Holton. "High sugar consumption could 'fuel' this process."

4. Carbohydrate-rich foods. Alright. Bread, pasta, crackers, muffins, and boxed cereals will only make your fibromyalgia symptoms worse. We know this won't win over many people. As long as you choose whole grains like quinoa, amaranth, and brown or wild rice, you can eat carbohydrates.

5. Glutamine. This is referred to as MSG (monosodium glutamate) and is used as a flavor enhancer.

Hydration

Hydration plays a crucial role in managing fibromyalgia symptoms and promoting overall health and well-being. While hydration alone may not directly treat fibromyalgia, maintaining adequate fluid intake can help alleviate some symptoms and support the body's physiological functions. Here's how hydration relates to fibromyalgia management:

1. Alleviating Symptoms:

Dehydration can exacerbate common symptoms of fibromyalgia, such as fatigue, headaches, and cognitive difficulties ("fibro fog"). By staying adequately hydrated, individuals with fibromyalgia may experience some relief from these symptoms. Proper hydration helps support optimal brain function, which can improve cognitive clarity and reduce fatigue.

2. Pain Management:

Dehydration can contribute to increased muscle stiffness and discomfort, which are hallmark symptoms of fibromyalgia. By ensuring sufficient hydration, individuals may experience better muscle function and reduced pain levels. Proper hydration also supports joint health and lubrication, potentially reducing pain associated with fibromyalgia.

3. Supporting Digestive Health:

Many individuals with fibromyalgia experience gastrointestinal symptoms such as irritable bowel syndrome (IBS) or abdominal discomfort. Hydration is essential for maintaining healthy digestion and bowel function. An adequate intake of fluids can help prevent constipation and promote regularity, thereby reducing gastrointestinal symptoms.

4. Enhancing Sleep Quality:

Proper hydration is linked to improved sleep quality, which is often disrupted in individuals with fibromyalgia. Dehydration can contribute to nighttime discomfort, such as dry mouth or muscle cramps, which may disrupt sleep patterns. By staying hydrated throughout the day, individuals may experience better sleep hygiene and improved overall sleep quality.

☐ Tips for Hydration in Fibromyalgia Management:

- Drink plenty of water throughout the day. Aim for at least eight 8-ounce glasses of water daily, but individual fluid needs may vary based on factors such as activity level, climate, and overall health.
- Incorporate hydrating foods into your diet, such as fruits and vegetables with high water content (e.g., cucumbers, watermelon, oranges).
- Limit caffeine and alcohol intake, as these substances can have diuretic effects and contribute to dehydration.
- Monitor urine color; pale yellow to clear urine generally indicates adequate hydration.
- Set reminders or use hydration tracking apps to ensure consistent fluid intake, especially if cognitive difficulties ("fibro fog") make it challenging to remember to drink water regularly.

While hydration is essential for fibromyalgia management, it's important to note that it is just one aspect of a comprehensive treatment approach. Individuals with fibromyalgia should work closely with their healthcare providers to develop personalized strategies for symptom management, which may include a combination of lifestyle modifications, medications, and therapies tailored to their specific needs.

Sleep Hygiene

If you visualize the symptoms of FM as a pie chart, sleep disorders would occupy approximately 25% of the pie. Even though many FM sufferers find it difficult to fall asleep, it's crucial to figure out how to get restorative sleep since that's when your body heals and your muscles mend. If you can conquer your sleep troubles, you will be a long way toward feeling better, and you will be in better shape to take on the day.

Make sure you've done everything possible to set up a sleep-friendly environment before thinking about taking sleep aids. Put another way, maintain proper sleeping habits.

☐ A PLACE FOR REST

Make sure your bedroom is a peaceful haven first. Remove any stuff that will distract you from your main objective—getting to sleep. This is not a time to sweep the toys under the bed for the kids. Ideally, do not use your bedroom as a place to socialize or as an office—this room should be a haven for relaxation, sex, and sleep.

Purchase the best mattress that fits your budget. If you are attempting to sleep on a bumpy, unpleasant mattress, and you can't afford a new one, try adding a mattress pad or a foam-rubber pad. Foam rubber is utilized in hospitals and is very comfortable to sleep on. There are no springs or hard areas pressing into your back and lower body, just foam that conforms to your shape. (Note: While foam rubber is fantastic for your back, it is a synthetic substance that may not be such a good idea to use if you have several chemical sensitivities.)

Many of our respondents recommended feather beds (fluffy, foldable mattresses, about three or four inches thick, that feel like heaven to rest on when laid over a mattress or foam pad). Spend as much as you can on your bedding—cotton or linen sheets and soft blankets with a down comforter is a perfect mix, both comfortable and sturdy. Don't layer the blankets too high. For optimal restorative sleep, your body temperature should be lower than it is during the day. So, try to keep your space cool and well ventilated.

"One can never have too many pillows," asserts Dr. Mick Tiegs, a chiropractor.

Your body is supported and braced by pillows when you sleep. Invest in enough,one beneath your knees to relieve weight off your back, and one to support your head and neck. Foam contour pillows are great for alignment and have been shown to enhance sleep quality. You might want to give them a try. Additionally, full-sized body pillows that support your entire body are offered.

☐ A SALIENT SETTLEMENT

As much as you can, rid your bedroom of toxins (this is especially crucial if you have several allergies or chemical sensitivities). Sheets and pillows composed of hypoallergenic natural fibers are available . Eliminate any furnishings made of synthetic materials as well. Particleboard and some paint types are examples of synthetic materials that release chemical vapors into the atmosphere. Older furniture that has had time to release its toxins or unpolished wood are the greatest options for creating a healthy atmosphere. The same is true with flooring; in addition to being chemically treated, synthetic carpets often include a variety of dirt, bacteria, and insects that trigger allergies. The healthiest flooring option for your bedroom is wood; but, if carpeting is your only alternative, consider sisal, lambswool, or throw rugs made of natural fiber that are easy to clean.

☐ CALM AND QUIET

Noisy background sounds make it hard to fall asleep, and unexpected noises frequently wake us up. You can reduce outside noise by adding plush carpets, thick curtains, or additional furniture. You can also try leaning a whole bookcase against the wall that bothers you. If you want to drown out the noise and fall asleep, you could wish to create a continuous background sound. One option that has the added benefit of cooling your space is a fan. Some people find that listening to the radio or even watching television helps them fall asleep. Many single folks find comfort and security in the companionship of their favorite late-night chat show or radio host. But don't forget to set the timer so your radio or TV will switch off; you never know when a different show can come on that will wake you up by stimulating your brain. You can also nod off with the aid of soothing noises or music. A feature of certain alarm clocks lets you choose the volume for when you wake up and go to sleep, so you can fall asleep to one sound and wake up to another. It is possible to find moderately priced alarm clocks with sound generators that may be programmed to softly wake you up in addition to lulling you to sleep. There are numerous sound effects to choose from, like rainstorms, breaking waves, and animals in the jungle. Another tool for blocking out noise is an earplug. They fit your ear perfectly and are reasonably priced.

☐ NIGHTLIGHT

While some find comfort in nightlights, others find it impossible to go asleep without them, most of us require darkness in order to doze off. If your windows let in too much light at night, you might want to get blackout liners or shades for your curtains (these are especially recommended if you live in Alaska or have a daytime sleep schedule). If the sun gets to you early in the morning, these liners come in handy too.

Our brains recognize darkness as the cue to go to sleep. Before the development of the electric light bulb, people followed the sun's cycle of rising and setting. Computers, TVs, and video games are examples of contemporary appliances that mess with our circadian cycles and cause sleeplessness. Aim to reduce the amount of light you are exposed to in the hours before bed. Before going to bed, avoid watching television or using the internet. Use a low-level reading light if you enjoy reading in bed. The best reading lights are those that clip onto a book since they are just dim enough to tell your brain when it's time to start calming down, yet they still allow you enough light to read without straining your eyes. If your companion enjoys staying up late reading when you want to go to sleep, you might want to recommend this to them. Another option is an eye mask, though you could have trouble falling asleep with something covering your eyes.

Remember to switch your illuminated alarm clock away from you, if it has one (or check to see if it has an off light). Not only do glowing digital clocks or glowing clock faces cause insomnia, but they also cause people to watch the seconds pass by, which exacerbates anxiety and makes it harder to fall asleep.

☐ FIELDS OF ELECTROMAGNETISM

You could wish to move your TV and radio alarm clock, or toss them away. To establish a healthy environment, many natural home specialists recommend eliminating items that emit electromagnetic fields (EMFs), which may cause tension and uneasiness in humans. Every electrical product emits electromagnetic radiation. Certain gadgets create unusually high levels of EMFs, such as conventional cathode ray computer monitors (Some people find that changing a CRT computer monitor with an LCD flat panel monitor can dramatically enhance their energy and attention).

Research is ambiguous regarding whether exposure to household EMFs causes harm to humans; nevertheless, eliminating as many electrical gadgets as possible clearly can't hurt and does provide a beautifully calming environment.

☐ NATURAL SLEEP AIDS

Introducing natural scents into the room can help lull you to sleep. Aromatherapist Jimm Harrison suggests lavender essential oil for its calming, stress-reducing effects. Chamomile, whether in essential oil form or in tea, can help soothe the body and induce sleep. Another effective herbal medicine that has been prized for thousands of years due to its calming properties is valerian root. You can assist restore your body's natural rhythm by taking a pill containing melatonin, a hormone that is produced naturally by our bodies.

Supplementing with melatonin can be beneficial, however the lowest effective dosage is recommended.

☐ A GOOD NIGHT'S SLEEP IS ESSENTIAL
Maintaining a consistent sleep schedule and eating your meals at the same time every day are two further suggested strategies for controlling your internal clock. Engaging in mild physical activity in the morning can also aid in your body's eventual relaxation. You need to unwind and minimize tension in order to get your body ready for sleep and to let go of the problems of the day. Try taking a warm bath and drinking a cup of hot milk. Tryptophan, an amino acid that the body uses to produce serotonin, is also present in milk and turkey, though a turkey sandwich might not sound too good right before bed. Hopefully, a few of these

suggestions will enable you to obtain the restorative sleep you so richly deserve.

greater). It's possible to find fairly priced alarm clocks with sound generators that may be programmed to assist you wake up and fall asleep.

CHAPTER SIX

HELPFUL TIPS FOR FIBROMYALGIA PATIENTS

- **Pain Prevention**

"Make sure your home has a well-defined path. Anything that could cause you to stumble should be moved aside. In the event that you have staircase, make sure you have a strong railing and that they are well-lit.

Nothing can aggravate your FM more than falling down stairs. To prevent your elbows from striking the wood, you should also wrap imitation lambswool across the chair's arms. From Lapwai, Idaho, Betty M.

If you find it difficult to balance in the bathroom and believe that slick flooring could be dangerous, you should think about installing grab bars and handrails. For installation and positioning instructions, visit a medical appliance store. Certain insurance providers will pay for this kind of gear. Another item to think about is a shower or bathtub seat. Everyone should have a bath mat, regardless matter whether they suffer from a chronic condition or not!
— Linda J. from Phoenix, AZ

"Be sure to dress appropriately for the weather because your body may interpret cold as pain. Remember to wear a hat; your head might lose up to 70% of your body heat.

— Mari S. from Seattle, WA

Employ an egg timer to monitor the amount of time you are spending on a project. This is especially useful if the task calls for extended standing or sitting. It's easy to lose track of time and wind up with back or neck spasms when a work is fun.

— Lois G. from Wisconsin's Stoughton

▢ Managing Pain

"I try taking a nice, hot bath or getting in my hot tub when I'm in pain." Last year, I bought a hot tub after realizing that the only time I was pain-free was in the water. The hydrotherapy aids in my discomfort, tension, and sleep. I count myself among the lucky people who own a hot tub, and I make time to use it at least three times a week. Usually on the weekends, I use it in the afternoon.

— Westfield, Massachusetts resident Susan G.

Avoid isolating oneself. Don't let your discomfort keep you inside four walls all the time. Save your energy for that evening with the grandchildren, go sit in the mall for thirty minutes, take a book to the neighborhood coffee shop, or sit in the front yard.

— Champaign, Illinois's Brenda S.

Participating in an art form that you are passionate about and that lifts your mind to a level where pain isn't as distracting is something I believe is vital. All people require beauty in their life, particularly those who have chronic suffering. Dancing makes me joyful, therefore when I dance, I don't feel my discomfort as much. Other art forms exist, of course, like painting or appreciating the paintings of others, theater, or music. Engaging in art that is captivating enough to take your mind off of your suffering and make you happy is the goal.

— Linda M. from Seattle, WA

"I consciously choose to show up for my own life because I've come to the realization that no matter where my body is or what I do, I will experience bodily agony! I still have moderate to severe chronic pain, but this insight led to a drastic paradigm change in which my life became the primary focus and the pain faded into the background.

— Seattle, Washington's Ellen J.

☐ Getting the Sleep You Require

I've turned my house into a safe haven for me because I live alone. Nobody has the right to interfere with my routine or "me time" when I'm not feeling well. Kim A. from Las Vegas, NV

"Weekdays or weekends, I often go to bed at the same hour every day. Getting enough sleep is a top priority for
me. I've improved my ability to pace myself. In the past, I would simply keep going until I was completely worn out. I don't do that anymore. Christine R. from Michigan's Sault Ste. Marie

"I make an effort to include my FM "down time" in my daily schedule." — Linda M.

❏ Your Power Source

"If I discover that I've overscheduled, I have to adjust my schedule and take a break. Since deadlines can be stressful, I try not to use them too much. I make a lot of effort to keep my deadlines flexible. Too many "Have To Dos" paralyze and overwhelm me. I even divide simple jobs into manageable chunks and concentrate on completing one little step at a time, sometimes spreading those small efforts over several days. Sally L., from Euless, TX

"I tackle things one step at a time. I try not to put myself under pressure with deadlines; instead, I set a goal and then take incremental steps, or larger steps if I can." — Happy Jack, Arizona's Katrina B. "Be truthful about your abilities and limitations, both to yourself and to other people. Never forget that only you truly understand how you are feeling and that only you are capable of caring for yourself. Even though your body may not be under your control, your mind is still under your power. — Shelbyville, Tennessee's Chandy W.

☐ Brain Fog

"To keep organized, I create lists." I always aim to finish the most difficult task first thing in the morning. I schedule my meals a week ahead of time to avoid having to worry about them every day.
— Candace Y. from California's Newport Beach

"Try recording your thoughts or feelings of brain fog the day before your outburst. Did you have a large pretzel or pizza? Do you have allergies?
- Journaling:
"I keep a symptom journal to track my progress." focusing on my treatment plan.
— Carver, Massachusetts resident Robin N.

"When I'm having a really rough day, I realize that I've been here before by looking back at my journal."
— Joan H., Canada's Victoria

Writing down your emotions can be rather healing. You are not required to write for publications, possess writing skills, or share your work with others unless you choose to. See if it helps, and give it a try sometime. — Linda M.

I keep a "gratitude journal," in which I list five or more items each day for which I am grateful. It makes it easier for me to change my attention from everything to be depressed about to all the little things I have every day to be thankful for. When I'm not feeling well, someone gets to interfere with my routine or "me time." — Sally L. Kim A. from Las Vegas, NV

Printed in Great Britain
by Amazon